CONTENTS

INTRODUCTION

The Optavia diet concept was introduced by the team behind Medifast, a famous meal replacement company. Following the Optavia program requires you to feed on low calorie and reduced carb foods. You will need a combination of packaged foods and homemade meals to lose weight effectively. If you don't enjoy cooking or you are a busy type, and you don't have enough time to cook your meals, the Optavia diet will be great for you as it doesn't require you to do prolonged cooking.

It is important to note that while Medifast does not require one-on-one coaching, the Optavia diet requires. Optavia diet enhances weight loss through branded products known as fueling while the homemade entrées are referred to as the Lean and Green meals. The fuelings are made up of over 60 items that are specifically low carbs but are high in probiotic cultures and Protein. The fuelings ultimately contain friendly bacteria that can help to boost gut health. They include; cookies, bars, puddings, shakes, soups, cereals, and pasta.

Looking at the listed foods, you might think they are quite high in carbs, that is understandable, but the fuelings are composed in such a way that they are lower in sugar and carbs than the traditional versions of the similar foods. The company does this by using small portion sizes and sugar substitutes. In furtherance to this, many of the fuelings are packed with soy protein isolate and whey protein powder. Those interested in the Optavia diet plan but are not interested or got no chance to cook are provided with pre-made low-carb meals by the company. These meals are referred to as Flavors of Home, and they can sufficiently replacing the Lean and Green Meals.

The company explicitly states that by working with its team of coaches and following the Optavia diet as required, you will achieve a "lifelong transformation, one healthy habit at a time."

Therefore, to record success with this diet plan, you have to stick to the fuelings which are supplemented by with veggie, meat, and healthy fat entrée daily, you will be full and nourished. Although you will be consuming low calories, you will not be losing a lot of muscle since you will be feeding on lots of fibre, protein, and other vital nutrients. Your calories as an adult will not exceed 800-1,000. You can lose 12 pounds in 12 weeks if you follow the optimal weight 5&1 plan option.

Since you will curb your carb intake while on this diet plan, you will naturally shed fat because the carb is the primary source of energy, therefore, if it is not readily available, the body finds a fat alternative, which implies that the body will have to break down your fats for energy and keep burning fat.

Summary: The Optavia diet is an idea of Medifast, and it comprises of pre-purchased portioned snacks and meals, low carb Lean and Green (homemade) meals, and continuous coaching that is based on facilitating fat and weight loss.

WHAT IS THE OPTAVIA DIET?

Optavia dieting is a practice aimed at reducing weight or maintaining one's current weight. It recommends eating a combination of processed food referred to as fuelings, and homemade meals (lean and green meals). It is believed that sticking to the brand's product (fuelings) and supplementing it with meat, veggies, and fat entrée every day; this will keep you full and adequately nourished. And there are no worries about losing muscles as you'll be eating a lot of protein and consuming few calories. And in this way, the individuals involved can lose about 12 pounds in just 12 weeks using the 5&1 optimal weight plan.

Put simply optavia diet is a program that focuses on lower calories and the reduction of carbohydrate meals. To do this effectively, it combines packed food called fuellings with homemade meals, thus encouraging loss of weight.

The name "Optavia" should sound like a new drug or eye-wear brand, but it is a weight loss program that has become famous thanks to the internet. Google named Optavia one of the hottest diets of 2018 in its year-end report, and Cake Boss Star Buddy Valastro said he lost weight thanks to this program.

"A lot of people demanded me how I managed to lose weight, so I just wanted to share that I used the Optavia program," he wrote on Instagram in June 2018.

I am not paid to say it, and it should be noted that I think everyone is different, and you should be on a diet doing that reflects you the most, but I am delighted with the results! ".

The diet is not a simple one: the program limits calories and advises its affiliates to buy "supplies" to lose weight. In fact, Optavia is a weight loss or maintenance program that recommends eating a mix of processed foods - called "supplies" - and homemade "lean green" meals.

The plan also recommends doing about 30 minutes of moderate intensity exercise a day.

Medifast's team has released a new product line under the OPTAVIA brand, with the same macronutrients as its original Medifast products. The company claims that by working with its coaches and following a diet that includes OPTAVIA products, "a permanent transformation" is achieved.

In detail, keep the brand products called "Fuelings" and supplement them with an appetizer of meat, vegetables, and healthy fats every day, you will be full and well-fed. Plus, you won't lose muscle because you'll be eating a lot of protein, fiber, and critical nutrients while consuming very few calories - about 800 to 1,000 for adults.

Customers lose around 12 pounds in 12 weeks with the Optimal Weight 5 & 1 plan.

Optavia adds a social support component access to a health coach who can answer questions and give encouragement.

How Does The Optavia Diet Work?

Most people follow the 5 & 1 program that incorporates 5 refills per day.

With this program, customers eat 5 of Optavia's "supplies" and 1 lean and green low-calorie homemade meal per day.

You can also choose more than 60 options, including smoothies, bars, soups, cookies, and pudding, including high-quality protein and 1 probiotic that the brand claims to aid digestive health. Your sixth daily meal (that you can eat at any time), is built around cooked lean protein, 3 servings of non-starchy vegetables, and healthy fats.

During the diet, you will work with Optavia trainers and be able to join a community to share your success. Once you've reached your weight goal, transitioning from the plan should be more comfortable as your old habits are replaced by healthier ones. Optavia offers a specific product line through its 3 and 3 plan for weight maintenance.

For people who want a more flexible and high-calorie diet, OPTAVIA suggests the 4 & 2 & 1 plan that incorporates 4 meals, 2 lean and green meals, and 1 healthy snack, like a baked potato serving fruit.

Optavia also sells specific programs for people with diabetes, nursing moms, the elderly and teenagers.

Benefits of Optavia Diet

1. Packaged products offer convenience

Optavia's smoothies, soups, and other meal replacement products are shipped to your door, providing a level of convenience that many other diets don't offer.

Even if you will need to purchase your ingredients for "lean and green" meals, Optavia's home delivery option for "supplies" helps a lot.

Once the products arrive, they are easy to prepare and make great takeaway meals.

2. Achieve rapid weight loss

Most healthy people need around 1,600-3,000 calories per day to maintain their weight. Limiting that amount to a minimum of 800 guarantees weight loss for most people.

Optavia's 5 & 1 plan is designed for rapid weight loss, making it a viable option for someone with a medical reason to lose weight fast.

3. Eliminate the guesswork

Some people say that the most challenging part of a diet is the mental effort to figure out what to eat each day or at each meal.

Optavia relieves the stress of meal planning and "decision fatigue" by offering users approved foods with "supplies" and guidelines for "lean and green" meals.

4. Offers social support

Social support is an essential component of the success of any weight loss program. Optavia's coaching program and group call ensure integrated encouragement and support for users.

Foods That Are Allowed

Many of the Optavia plans include its "supplies," like bars, smoothies, cookies, cereals and some savory options, such as soup and mashed potatoes. These processed foods often list soy or whey protein as their first ingredient. Lean, green meals complement the rest of the diet, which you purchase and prepare yourself.

These include:

- 5-7 ounces of cooked lean protein like egg white, chicken, fish, soy;
- 3 servings of non-starchy vegetables like cucumbers, lettuce, celery;
- 2 servings of healthy fats like olives, olive oil, avocado.

Based on the Optavia diet plan you choose; you will eat 2 to 5 prepackaged replacement meals per day.

You will prepare and eat 1 to 3 of your low-calorie meals, that should be mostly lean protein and non-starchy vegetables.

While no food is technically prohibited in the diet, many (such as sweets) are discouraged.

Free-range turkey

Always check the label and choose a lean turkey cut that complies with Optavia's guidelines for your sixth meal.

Pumpkin seeds

Put salt and pepper to give it flavor. You can also mix pumpkin seeds in a salad.

Grilled shrimp

With this lean protein, you can create many varieties of meals. Thread a few skewers and arrange them on the grill or season the shrimp with Cajun spices and serve with grilled peppers and zucchini on the side.

Cucumbers

The Optavia diet requires non-starchy vegetables for the sixth daily meal. Cucumbers may work for you, or you can snack on celery sticks.

Tuna

If you travel a lot, this light meal does not require any preparation time. Take a can of tuna and stir with freshly squeezed lemon juice, chopped celery, and olives.

Vegetable noodles

Make vegetarian zucchini "noodles" for a low-carb alternative to pasta as part of your lean, green meal.

Lean Meals

The "lean and green" meals you prepare should incorporate a 5 to 7 ounce serving of cooked lean protein.

Optavia differentiates between lean, leaner, and leanest protein sources.

I'll give you some examples to distinguish them:

Lean: salmon, lamb or pork chops;

Leaner: swordfish or chicken breast;

Leanest: cod, shrimp and egg whites.

Green Meal

In the Optavia's 5 & 1 program, you can add 2 non-starchy vegetables and protein to your lean and green meal.

Vegetables are broken down into lower, moderate, and higher carb categories, with the following examples:

Low carb: green salad;

Moderate carbohydrates: cauliflower or summer squash;

Higher carbohydrates: broccoli or peppers.

Healthy fats

Beyond lean protein and non-starchy vegetables, a lean and green meal can be made with 2 servings of healthy fats like olive or nut oil, flax-seed, or avocado.

Low-fat dairy products, fresh fruit and whole grains

When people have achieved their desired weight loss through meal replacements, lean proteins, and non-starchy vegetables, they can switch to a plan to maintain their weight.

In Optavia's weight maintenance plans, users can start reintroducing other foods. Low-fat dairy, fruit and whole grains are incorporated in Optavia's 3 & 3 and 4 & 2 & 1 weight maintenance plans.

POSSIBLE DOWNSIDES OF THE OPTAVIA DIET

Although the Optavia diet is an effective weight-loss tool, it has some potential disadvantages. Some of its downsides are:

Meagre calorie consumption

- The Optavia diet only room for only 800-1,200 calories consumed daily while on the 5&1 plan, which is very low for an adult consuming more than 2,000 calories before then.
- Even though the low-calorie intake can significantly result in weight loss, it can also lead to muscle loss.
- Studies have shown that low-calorie diets can lead to frequent hunger and cravings, which can make adhering to the diet plan more difficult.

It can be challenging to stick with

- The 5&1 plan of the Optavia diet program includes five prepackaged fuelings and 1 Lean and Green meal (low carb) only. This shows that the program has restricted food options and low-calorie count; hence, it can be difficult to stick by it.
- Since the food options are restricted and not what you are used to, you can get tired along the line while on the program, and as such, you can easily develop cravings for other foods and cheat on the diet.
- Even though the maintenance plan is not as restrictive as the other two control plans, it also depends mainly on fuelings.

The Optavia Diet program can be Expensive.

The Optavia diet can be costly regardless of which of the plan you chose. An average of 3 weeks' worth of Optavia fuelings, which can be in the region of 120 servings while on the 5&1 plan can cost between $350-$450. However, this cost will also include the coaching for that period, but it does not cover the cost of groceries for the recommended Lean and Green meals.

How Nutritious is Optavia Diet

Below is the breakdown comparison of the nutritional content of meals on the Optavial Weight 5&1 Plan and the federal government's 2015 Dietary Guidelines for Americans.

Note that since lean and green meals vary, the figures given below are estimates. The diet figures are retrieved from OPTAVIA:

	Optimal Weight 5&1 Plan	Federal Government Recommendation
Calories	800-1,000	Men 19-25: 2,800 26-45: 2,600 46-65: 2,400 65+: 2,200 Women 19-25: 2,200 26-50: 2,000 51+: 1,800
Total fat % of Calorie Intake	20%	20%-35%
Saturated Fat % of Calorie Intake	3%-5%	Less than 10%
Trans Fat % of Calorie Intake	0%	N/A
Total Carbohydrates % of Calorie Intake	40%	45%-65%
Sugars (Total except as noted)	10%-20%	N/A
Fiber	25 g – 30 g	Men 19-30: 34 g. 31-50: 31 g. 51+: 28 g. Women 19-30: 28 g. 31-50: 25 g. 51+: 22 g.
Protein % of Calorie Intake	40%	10%-35%

Sodium	Under 2,300 mg	Under 2,300 mg.
Potassium	Average 3,000 mg	At least 4,700 mg.
Calcium	1,000 mg – 1,200 mg	Men 1,000 mg. Women 19-50: 1,000 mg. 51+: 1,200 mg.
Vitamin B-12	2.4 mcg	2.4 mcg.
Vitamin D	20 mcg – 50 mcg.	15 mcg

Note that: g = gram, mg = milligram, mcg = microgram

Do's & Don'ts of the Optavia Diet

The Optavia diet plan has some guidelines, especially in food consumption that must be adhered to if you wish to record a significant success with the diet plan.

Recommended Foods to eat

The foods you are liable to eat while on the 5&1 plan are the 5 Optavia fuellings and 1 Lean and Green meal daily. The meals consist mainly of healthy fats, lean protein, and low carb vegetables, and there is a recommendation for only two servings of fatty fish every week. Some beverages and low carb condiments are also allowed in small proportions.

The foods that are allowed for the Lean and Green meals are:

- Fish and Shellfish: Trout, tuna, halibut, salmon, crab, scallops, lobster, shrimp.
- Meat: Lean beef, lamb, chicken, game meats, turkey, tenderloin or pork chop, ground meat (must be 85% lean at least)
- Vegetable oils: walnut, flaxseed, olive oil, and canola
- Eggs: Whole eggs, egg beaters, egg whites
- Additional healthy fats: reduced-fat margarine, walnuts, pistachios, almonds, avocado, olives, low carb salad dressings.
- Soy Products: Tofu
- Sugar-free beverages: unsweetened almond milk, coffee, tea, water
- Sugar-free snacks: gelatin, mints, popsicles, gum
- Low carb vegetables: celery, mushrooms, cauliflower, zucchini, peppers, jicama, spinach, cucumbers, cabbage, eggplant, broccoli, spaghetti squash, collard greens
- Seasonings and Condiments: lemon juice, yellow mustard, salsa, zero-calorie sweeteners, barbecue sauce, cocktail sauce, dried herbs, salt, spices, lime juice, soy sauce, sugar-free syrup, ½ teaspoons only of ketchup.

Summary: The Optavia 5&1 plan homemade meals consist mainly of low carb veggies, lean proteins, and a few healthy fats. It allows only low carb beverages like unsweetened almond milk, water, tea, and coffee.

Foods That Are Not Allowed

Apart from the carbs contained in the prepackaged Optavia fuelings, most carb-containing beverages and foods are not allowed while you are on the 5&1 Plan. Some fats are also banned as well as all fried foods.

Below are the foods you must avoid except they are included in your fuelings:

- Refined grains: pasta, pancakes, crackers, cookies, pastries, white bread, biscuits, flour tortillas, white rice, cakes
- Fried foods: Fish, vegetables, shellfish, meats, sweets like pastries
- Whole fat dairy: cheese, milk, yoghurt
- Certain fats: coconut oil, butter, solid shortening
- Sugar-sweetened beverages: fruit juice, soda, energy drinks, sports drinks, sweet tea
- Alcohol: All varieties

The foods below are banned while on the 5&1 plan but are added for the 6-week transition phase and with no restriction during the 3&3 Plan:

- Fruit: All fresh fruit
- Whole grains: high fibre breakfast cereal, whole grain bread, whole-wheat pasta, brown rice
- Starch vegetables: corn, white potatoes, sweet potatoes, peas
- Low-fat or fat-free dairy: milk, yoghurt, cheese
- Legumes: Beans, peas, lentils, soybeans

Note that during the six weeks' transition phase, and while on the 3&3 plan, you are advised to eat more berries if you must take fruits as they contain lower carbs.

SHOPPING LIST FOR OPTAVIA DIET

1. Breakfast

7 ounce Spelt Flour
1 cup Coconut Milk
1/2 cup Alkaline Water
2 tbsps. Grapeseed Oil
1/2 cup Agave
1/2 cup Blueberries
1/4 tsp. Sea Moss
1 cup raspberry
1/2 teaspoon restrained oil
1/2 cup sun-dried tomatoes
2 cups of spinach
1/2 spoon drops of zaatar spices
10 eggs
1/2 cup Feta cheese
salt and pepper
Canola oil
1/2 Cup Coarse cornmeal
1/2 tablespoon red pepper
1/4 baking soda
1 1/2 Cup Flour for all purposes is divided
Kosher salt and freshly ground black pepper
1 12 oz can drink beer in style
1 code and skin without skin
1 large cup of peeled and spread shrimp
16 percentiles, shake
1 lemon sliced with cedar wedge
Tartar sauce, mignon, chimichurri, hot sauce, and malt vinegar, for cedar
1/2 Cup Mayonnaise
2 teaspoons, pickled, chopped or pureed
1 tablespoon fresh lemon juice
1 tablespoon three-quarter pants
1 tablespoon mustard
Kosher salt

2. Mains

1-pound rib eye steak
1 teaspoon salt
1 teaspoon cayenne pepper
½ teaspoon chili flakes
3 tablespoon cream
1 teaspoon olive oil
1 teaspoon lemongrass
1 tablespoon butter
1 teaspoon garlic powder

3. Sides

4 zucchinis sliced
1 ½ cups parmesan; grated
¼ cup parsley; chopped.
1 egg; whisked
1 egg white; whisked
½ tsp. garlic powder
Cooking spray
Fuelings recipes
2 eggs
1/2 cup fresh blueberries
1 cup heavy cream
2 cups almond flour
1/4 tsp lemon zest
1/2 tsp lemon extract
1 tsp baking powder
5 drops stevia
1/4 cup butter

4. Seafood

¼ cup chopped fresh cilantro
½ cup seeded and finely chopped plum tomato
1 cup peeled and finely chopped mango
1 lime cut into wedges
1 tablespoon chipotle Chile powder
1 tablespoon safflower oil
1/3 cup finely chopped red onion
10 tablespoon fresh lime juice, divided
4 6-oz boneless, skinless cod fillets
5 tablespoon dried unsweetened shredded coconut
8 pcs of 6-inch tortillas

5. Lean and Green

14 ounces of jumbo cooked shrimp, peeled and deveined; chopped
4 ½ ounces of avocado, diced
1 ½ cup of tomato, diced
¼ cup of chopped green onion
¼ cup of jalapeno with the seeds removed, diced fine
1 teaspoon of olive oil
2 tablespoons of lime juice
1/8 teaspoon of salt
1 tablespoon of chopped cilantro

6. Snacks

15 ounces canned white beans, drained and rinsed
6 ounces canned artichoke hearts, drained and quartered
4 garlic cloves, minced
1 tablespoon basil, chopped
2 tablespoons olive oil
Juice of ½ lemon
Zest of ½ lemon, grated
Salt and black pepper

7. Smoothies

1 tsp chia seeds
½ cup unsweetened coconut milk
1 avocado
3 quartered frozen Burro Bananas
1-1/2 cups of Homemade Coconut Milk
1/4 cup of Walnuts
1 teaspoon of Sea Moss Gel
1 teaspoon of Ground Ginger
1 teaspoon of Soursop Leaf Powder
1 handful of Kale

8. Starches and Grains

2 tablespoons extra-virgin olive oil
1 onion
4 cups fresh baby spinach
1 garlic clove, minced
Zest of 1 orange
Juice of 1 orange
1 cup unsalted vegetable broth
2 cups cooked brown rice
Soup and Salad
For the walnuts
2 tablespoons butter
¼ cup sugar or honey
1 cup walnut pieces
½ teaspoon kosher salt
3 tablespoons extra-virgin olive oil
1½ tablespoons champagne vinegar
1½ tablespoons Dijon mustard
¼ teaspoon kosher salt
1 head red leaf lettuce, shredded into pieces
3 heads endive
2 apples
1 (8-ounce) Camembert wheel

9. Meat

1 lb beef chuck roast
1 fresh lime juice
1 garlic clove
1 teaspoon chili powder
2 cups lemon-lime soda
1/2 teaspoon salt

10. Fast and Cheap

2 cups mayonnaise
6 plum tomatoes, seeded and finely chopped
1/4 cup ketchup
1/4 cup lemon juice
2 cups seedless red and/or green grapes, halved
1 tablespoon. Worcestershire sauce
2 lbs. peeled and deveined cooked large shrimp
2 celery ribs, finely chopped
3 tablespoons. minced fresh tarragon or 3 teaspoon dried tarragon
salt and 1/4 teaspoon pepper
shredded 2 of cups romaine
papaya or 1/2 cup peeled chopped mango
parsley or minced chives

BREAKFAST RECIPES

11. Alkaline Blueberry Spelt Pancakes

Preparation Time: 6 minutes
Cooking Time: 20 minutes
Servings: 3
INGREDIENTS:

- 2 cups Spelt Flour
- 1 cup Coconut Milk
- 1/2 cup Alkaline Water
- 2 tbsps. Grapeseed Oil
- 1/2 cup Agave
- 1/2 cup Blueberries
- 1/4 tsp. Sea Moss

DIRECTIONS:

1. Mix the spelt flour, agave, grapeseed oil, hemp seeds, and the sea moss together in a bowl.
2. Add in 1 cup of hemp milk and alkaline water to the mixture, until you get the consistency mixture you like.
3. Crimp the blueberries into the batter.
4. Heat the skillet to moderate heat then lightly coat it with the grapeseed oil.
5. Pour the batter into the skillet then let them cook for approximately 5 minutes on every side.
6. Serve and Enjoy.

NUTRITION: Calories: 203 kcal Fat: 1.4g Carbs: 41.6g Proteins: 4.8g

12. Alkaline Blueberry Muffins

Preparation Time: 5 Minutes
Cooking Time: 20 minutes
Servings: 3
INGREDIENTS:

- 1 cup Coconut Milk
- 3/4 cup Spelt Flour
- 3/4 Teff Flour
- 1/2 cup Blueberries
- 1/3 cup Agave
- 1/4 cup Sea Moss Gel
- 1/2 tsp. Sea Salt
- Grapeseed Oil

DIRECTIONS:

1. Adjust the temperature of the oven to 365 degrees.
2. Grease 6 regular-size muffin cups with muffin liners.
3. In a bowl, mix together sea salt, sea moss, agave, coconut milk, and flour gel until they are properly blended.
4. You then crimp in blueberries.
5. Coat the muffin pan lightly with the grapeseed oil.
6. Pour in the muffin batter.
7. Bake for at least 30 minutes until it turns golden brown.
8. Serve.

NUTRITION: Calories: 160 kcal Fat: 5g Carbs: 25g Proteins: 2g

13. Crunchy Quinoa Meal

Preparation Time: 5 minutes
Cooking Time: 25 minutes
Servings: 2
INGREDIENTS:

- 3 cups coconut milk
- 1 cup rinsed quinoa
- 1/8 tsp. ground cinnamon
- 1 cup raspberry
- 1/2 cup chopped coconuts

DIRECTIONS:

1. In a saucepan, pour milk and bring to a boil over moderate heat.
2. Add the quinoa to the milk and then bring it to a boil once more.
3. You then let it simmer for at least 15 minutes on medium heat until the milk is reduced.
4. Stir in the cinnamon then mix properly.
5. Cover it then cook for 8 minutes until the milk is completely absorbed.
6. Add the raspberry and cook the meal for 30 seconds.
7. Serve and enjoy.

NUTRITION: Calories: 271 kcal Fat: 3.7g Carbs: 54g Proteins: 6.5g

14. Coconut Pancakes

Preparation Time: 5 minutes
Cooking Time: 15 minutes
Servings: 4
INGREDIENTS:

- 1 cup coconut flour
- 2 tbsps. arrowroot powder
- 1 tsp. baking powder
- 1 cup coconut milk
- 3 tbsps. coconut oil

DIRECTIONS:

1. In a medium container, mix in all the dry ingredients.
2. Add the coconut milk and 2 tbsps. of the coconut oil then mix properly.
3. In a skillet, melt 1 tsp. of coconut oil.
4. Pour a ladle of the batter into the skillet then swirl the pan to spread the batter evenly into a smooth pancake.
5. Cook it for like 3 minutes on medium heat until it becomes firm.
6. Turn the pancake to the other side then cook it for another 2 minutes until it turns golden brown.
7. Cook the remaining pancakes in the same process.
8. Serve.

NUTRITION: Calories: 377 kcal Fat: 14.9g Carbs: 60.7g Protein: 6.4g

15. Quinoa Porridge

Preparation Time: 5 minutes
Cooking Time: 25 minutes
Servings: 2
INGREDIENTS:

- 2 cups coconut milk
- 1 cup rinsed quinoa
- 1/8 tsp. ground cinnamon
- 1 cup fresh blueberries

DIRECTIONS:

1. In a saucepan, boil the coconut milk over high heat.
2. Add the quinoa to the milk then bring the mixture to a boil.
3. You then let it simmer for 15 minutes on medium heat until the milk is reduces.
4. Add the cinnamon then mix it properly in the saucepan.
5. Cover the saucepan and cook for at least 8 minutes until milk is completely absorbed.
6. Add in the blueberries then cook for 30 more seconds.
7. Serve.

NUTRITION: Calories: 271 kcal Fat: 3.7g Carbs: 54g Protein:6.5g

16. Amaranth Porridge

Preparation Time: 5 minutes
Cooking Time: 30 minutes
Servings: 2.
INGREDIENTS:

- 2 cups coconut milk
- 2 cups alkaline water
- 1 cup amaranth
- 2 tbsps. coconut oil
- 1 tbsp. ground cinnamon

DIRECTIONS:

1. In a saucepan, mix in the milk with water then boil the mixture.
2. You stir in the amaranth then reduce the heat to medium.
3. Cook on the medium heat then simmer for at least 30 minutes as youstir it occasionally.
4. Turn off the heat.
5. Add in cinnamon and coconut oil then stir.
6. Serve.

NUTRITION: Calories: 434 kcal Fat: 35g Carbs: 27g Protein: 6.7g

17. Banana Barley Porridge

Preparation Time: 15 minutes
Cooking Time: 5 minutes
Servings: 2
INGREDIENTS:

- 1 cup divided unsweetened coconut milk
- 1 small peeled and sliced banana
- 1/2 cup barley
- 3 drops liquid stevia
- 1/4 cup chopped coconuts

DIRECTIONS:

1. In a bowl, properly mix barley with half of the coconut milk and stevia.
2. Cover the mixing bowl then refrigerate for about 6 hours.
3. In a saucepan, mix the barley mixture with coconut milk.
4. Cook for about 5 minutes on moderate heat.
5. Then top it with the chopped coconuts and the banana slices.
6. Serve.

NUTRITION: Calories: 159kcal Fat: 8.4g Carbs: 19.8g Proteins: 4.6g

18. Zucchini Muffins

Preparation Time: 10 minutes
Cooking Time: 25 minutes
Servings: 16
INGREDIENTS:

- 1 tbsp. ground flaxseed
- 3 tbsps. alkaline water
- 1/4 cup walnut butter
- 3 medium over-ripe bananas
- 2 small grated zucchinis
- 1/2 cup coconut milk
- 1 tsp. vanilla extract
- 2 cups coconut flour
- 1 tbsp. baking powder
- 1 tsp. cinnamon
- 1/4 tsp. sea salt

DIRECTIONS:

1. Tune the temperature of your oven to 375ºF.
2. Grease the muffin tray with the cooking spray.
3. In a bowl, mix the flaxseed with water.
4. In a glass bowl, mash the bananas then stir in the remaining ingredients.
5. Properly mix and then divide the mixture into the muffin tray.
6. Bake it for 25 minutes.
7. Serve.

NUTRITION: Calories: 127 kcal Fat: 6.6g Carbs: 13g Protein: 0.7g

19. Millet Porridge

Preparation Time: 10 minutes
Cooking Time: 20 minutes
Servings: 2
INGREDIENTS:

- Sea salt
- 1 tbsp. finely chopped coconuts
- 1/2 cup unsweetened coconut milk
- 1/2 cup rinsed and drained millet
- 1-1/2 cups alkaline water
- 3 drops liquid stevia

DIRECTIONS:

1. Sauté the millet in a non-stick skillet for about 3 minutes.
2. Add salt and water then stir.
3. Let the meal boil then reduce the amount of heat.
4. Cook for 15 minutes then add the remaining ingredients. Stir.
5. Cook the meal for 4 extra minutes.
6. Serve the meal with toping of the chopped nuts.

NUTRITION: Calories: 219 kcal Fat: 4.5g Carbs: 38.2g Protein: 6.4g

20. Jackfruit Vegetable Fry

Preparation Time: 5 minutes
Cooking Time: 5 minutes
Servings: 6
INGREDIENTS:

- 2 finely chopped small onions
- 2 cups finely chopped cherry tomatoes
- 1/8 tsp. ground turmeric
- 1 tbsp. olive oil
- 2 seeded and chopped red bell peppers
- 3 cups seeded and chopped firm jackfruit
- 1/8 tsp. cayenne pepper
- 2 tbsps. chopped fresh basil leaves
- Salt

DIRECTIONS:

1. In a greased skillet, sauté the onions and bell peppers for about 5 minutes.
2. Add the tomatoes then stir.
3. Cook for 2 minutes.
4. Then add the jackfruit, cayenne pepper, salt, and turmeric.
5. Cook for about 8 minutes.
6. Garnish the meal with basil leaves.
7. Serve warm.

NUTRITION: Calories: 236 kcal Fat: 1.8g Carbs: 48.3g Protein: 7g

21. Zucchini Pancakes

Preparation Time: 15 minutes
Cooking Time: 8 minutes
Servings: 8
INGREDIENTS:

- 12 tbsps. alkaline water
- 6 large grated zucchinis
- Sea salt
- 4 tbsps. ground Flax Seeds
- 2 tsps. olive oil
- 2 finely chopped jalapeño peppers
- 1/2 cup finely chopped scallions

DIRECTIONS:

1. In a bowl, mix together water and the flax seeds then set it aside.
2. Pour oil in a large non-stick skillet then heat it on medium heat.
3. The add the black pepper, salt, and zucchini.
4. Cook for 3 minutes then transfer the zucchini into a large bowl.
5. Add the flax seed and the scallion's mixture then properly mix it.
6. Preheat a griddle then grease it lightly with the cooking spray.
7. Pour 1/4 of the zucchini mixture into griddle then cook for 3 minutes.
8. Flip the side carefully then cook for 2 more minutes.
9. Repeat the procedure with the remaining mixture in batches.
10. Serve.

NUTRITION: Calories: 71 kcal Fat: 2.8g Carbs: 9.8g Protein: 3.7g

22. Squash Hash

Prep Time: 2 minutes
Cooking Time: 10 minutes
Servings: 2
INGREDIENTS:

- 1 tsp. onion powder
- 1/2 cup finely chopped onion
- 2 cups spaghetti squash
- 1/2 tsp. sea salt

DIRECTIONS:

1. Using paper towels, squeeze extra moisture from spaghetti squash.
2. Place the squash into a bowl then add the salt, onion, and the onion powder.
3. Stir properly to mix them.
4. Spray a non-stick cooking skillet with cooking spray then place it over moderate heat.
5. Add the spaghetti squash to pan.
6. Cook the squash for about 5 minutes.
7. Flip the hash browns using a spatula.
8. Cook for 5 minutes until the desired crispness is reached.
9. Serve.

NUTRITION: Calories: 44 kcal Fat: 0.6g Carbs: 9.7g Protein: 0.9g

23. Hemp Seed Porridge

Preparation Time: 5 minutes
Cooking Time: 5 minutes
Servings: 6
INGREDIENTS:

- 3 cups cooked hemp seed
- 1 packet Stevia
- 1 cup coconut milk

DIRECTIONS:

1. In a saucepan, mix the rice and the coconut milk over moderate heat for about 5 minutes as you stir it constantly.
2. Remove the pan from the burner then add the Stevia. Stir.
3. Serve in 6 bowls.
4. Enjoy.

NUTRITION: Calories: 236 kcal Fat: 1.8g Carbs: 48.3g Protein: 7g

24. Pumpkin Spice Quinoa

Preparation Time: 10 minutes
Cook Time: 0 minutes
Servings: 2
INGREDIENTS:

- 1 cup cooked quinoa
- 1 cup unsweetened coconut milk
- 1 large mashed banana
- 1/4 cup pumpkin puree
- 1 tsp. pumpkin spice
- 2 tsps. chia seeds

DIRECTIONS:

1. In a container, mix all the ingredients.
2. Seal the lid then shake the container properly to mix.
3. Refrigerate overnight.
4. Serve.

NUTRITION: Calories: 212 kcal Fat: 11.9g Carbs: 31.7g Protein: 7.3g

25. Easy, healthy Greek Salmon Salad

Preparation Time:10 minutes
Cooking Time:8 minutes
Servings:4
INGREDIENTS:

- ¼ cup olive oil
- 3 tablespoons red wine vinegar
- 2 tablespoons freshly crush lemon juice (from 1 lemon)
- 1 clove of garlic, chopped
- ¾ teaspoon dried oregano
- 1/2 teaspoon Kosar salt
- ¼ teaspoon fresh black pepper
- One finely chopped red onion
- A cup of cold water
- 4 (6 oz) salmon fillets, peeled
- 2 medium-sized Korean salads, such as Boston or Bibb (about 1 kilogram), broken into bite-size pieces
- 2 medium-sized tomatoes, cut into 1-inch pieces
- 1 medium English cucumber, quadrilateral and then cut into 1/2-inch pieces
- ½ cup of half-length Kalamata olives
- 4 oz Feta Cheese, minced (about 1 cup)

DIRECTIONS:

1. In the middle of the oven arrange a shelf and heat to 425 degrees Fahrenheit. While the oven is warming, marinate the salmon and soften the onion (instructions below).
2. Put the olive oil, vinegar, lemon juice, garlic, oregano, salt and pepper in a large bowl, then transfer three tablespoons of vinegar large enough into a baking dish to keep all the salmon chunks in one layer. Add the salmon, lightly rotate a few times to wrap evenly in the wings. Cover the fridge. Pour the onion and water into a small bowl and set aside 10 minutes to make the onion stronger. Drain and release the liquid.
3. Discover the salmon and grill for 8 to 12 minutes until they are cooked and lightly fried. Thermometer instant read in the middle of the thickest tab should record 120 degrees Fahrenheit to 130 degrees Fahrenheit for the rare medium or 135 degrees Fahrenheit to 145 degrees Fahrenheit. The total time of the cooking depends on the thickness of the salmon, depending on the thickest portion of the fillet. It Al depends on the salad.
4. Add the salad, tomatoes, cucumbers, olives, and red onion to the Gina Vine bowl and salt to combine. Divide into four plates or shallow bowl. When the salmon is ready, place one fillet over each salad. Sprinkle with feta and serve quickly.

NUTRITION: Calories: 351 Total fat: 4g Cholesterol: 94mg Fiber: 2g Protein: 12g Sodium: 327mg

26. Mediterranean Pepper

Preparation Time:5 minutes
Cooking Time:20 minutes
Servings:4
INGREDIENTS:

- 1/2 teaspoon restrained oil 1/2 cup sun-dried tomatoes
- 2 cups of spinach (fresh or frozen)
- 1/2 spoon drops of zaatar spices
- 10 eggs, screaming
- 1/2 cup Feta cheese
- 1-2 tablespoons
- salt and pepper

DIRECTIONS:

1. At 350 degrees Farenheit, firstly preheat the oven
2. Heat a cast-iron boiler over medium heat. Add the olive oil and peas, slowly and slowly cooking until you want to release the liquid and start to brown and brown. Then, sauté the sun-dried tomatoes with a little reserved oil, spinach and zucchini, and cook for 2-3 minutes until the spinach is crushed.
3. When the spinach has faded, pour the vegetable mixture evenly into the cast iron fish and then add the boiled eggs, turning the pan so that the eggs cover the vegetables evenly. Bake on medium heat until the eggs start about halfway through. Pour the eggs and vegetables with the spatula into the pan, leave the eggs to cook until the frittata is placed.
4. When the eggs are almost half cooked, add the Feta cheese and spoon the horseradish sauce on top and dust with salt and pepper. Remove the cast iron from the oven and place it in the middle rack in the oven. Bake until cooked on the ferrite, will take about five minutes.
5. Bring out from the oven and let it cool slightly. For cedar, cut or square the pie and pour with a pan.

NUTRITION: Calories: 311 Total fat: 4g Cholesterol: 84mg Fiber: 2g Protein: 12g Sodium: 357mg

27. Black Beans and Sweet Potato Tacos

Preparation Time:10 minutes
Cooking Time:30 minutes
Servings:6
INGREDIENTS:

- 1 lb. sweet potato (about 2 medium teaspoons), skin cut and cut into 1/2-inch pieces
- Divide into 2 tablespoons of olive oil
- 1 tablespoon Kosar salt, divided
- ¼ teaspoon fresh black pepper on large white or yellow onion, finely chopped
- 2 teaspoons of red pepper
- 1 cumin with a teaspoon
- 1 (15 oz.) can be black beans, drained and drained
- Cup of water
- ¼ cup freshly chopped garlic
- 12 pcs. Corn
- To Servings: guacamole
- Sliced cheese or feta cheese (optional)
- Wood Wedge

DIRECTIONS:

1. In the oven, set out a shelf in the middle and place to 425 degrees Fahrenheit. Set a big sheet of aluminum foil on the work surface. Collect the tortillas from the top and wrap them completely in foil. Put it aside
2. Put sweet potatoes on a small baking sheet. Mix with one tablespoon oil and sprinkle with 1/2 teaspoon salt and 1/4 teaspoon black pepper. Discard to mix and play in one layer. Fry for 20 minutes. Sprinkle the potatoes with a flat lid and set aside until a corner of the oven is clear.
3. Put the foil wrapping in the empty space and continue to cook for about 10 minutes until the sweet potatoes are browned and stained and the seasonings are heated. Also, cook the beans.
4. You then heat one tablespoon remaining in a large skillet over low heat. Put the onion and cook, occasionally stirring, until translucent, about 3 minutes. Mix the pepper powder, cumin, and 1/2 teaspoon salt. Add the beans and water.
5. Shield the pan and reduce the heat to low heat. Cook for 5 minutes, then slice and use the back of the fork to chop the beans a little, about half of the total. If there is still water in the vessel, stir the exposed mixture for about 30 seconds until evaporated.
6. Peel the sweet potatoes and add the cantaloupe to the black beans and mix. If used, fill the yolk with a mixture of black beans and top with guacamole and cheese. Serve with lime wedges.

NUTRITION: Calories: 251 Total fat: 4g Cholesterol: 94mg Fiber: 2g Protein: 15g Sodium: 329mg

28. Seafood Cooked from Beer

Preparation Time:30 minutes
Cooking Time: 1 hour
Servings:8
INGREDIENTS:
Seafood:

- Canola oil for roasting
- 1/2 Cup Coarse cornmeal
- 1/2 tablespoon red pepper
- 1/4 baking soda
- 1 1/2 Cup Flour for all purposes is divided
- Kosher salt and freshly ground black pepper
- 1 12 oz can drink beer in style
- 1 code and skin without skin, cut into 8 strips
- 1 large cup (number 25/25) of peeled and spread shrimp (remaining tail)
- 16 percentiles, shake
- 1 lemon sliced with cedar wedge
- Tartar sauce, mignon, chimichurri, hot sauce, and malt vinegar, for cedar

Sos tartar:

- 1/2 Cup Mayonnaise
- 2 teaspoons, pickled, chopped or pureed
- 1 tablespoon fresh lemon juice
- 1 tablespoon three-quarter pants
- 1 tablespoon mustard
- Kosher salt and freshly ground black pepper
- 1/2 Cup Red wine vinegar
- 1 small rest, finely chopped
- Kosher salt and freshly ground black pepper
- chimichurri:
- 1/2 Cup Fresh parsley on a flat-leaf
- 1/4 Cup White wine vinegar
- 2 tablespoons olive oil
- 2 cloves of minced garlic
- 1 stem, seeds and mincemeat
- 1 tablespoon fresh oregano, chopped
- Sare Kosar

DIRECTIONS:

1. Heat 1 1/2-inch oil in a large Dutch oven over medium heat at 375 degrees F (deep-fried temperature with a thermometer).
2. Meanwhile, chop corn, bell pepper, baking soda, 1 cup of flour, 1/2 teaspoon salt, and 1/2 teaspoon pepper in a bowl. Add the broth and the phloem to mix.
3. Put 1/2 cup of the remaining flour in a bowl. Add salt, pepper and the fish, shrimps, shells, and lemon slices and serve little.
4. Work several pieces at once, remove the seafood and the lemons from the flour, shake too much, and drain the dough and allow the excess drops to return to the container. Carefully add the hot oil, being careful not to overload the pot. Roast golden brown and cook for 1 to 2 minutes. Transfer to a sheet of paper towel — season with salt.
5. Make the tartar sauce: mayonnaise, pickled or mixed the cloves, and pour the lemon juice, pepper, and mustard whole in a bowl. Season with Kosar salt and freshly ground pepper, feel free to add more lemon juice. Face 2/3 glass.
6. To Make Mignonette: add red wine vinegar and finely minced mustard in a bowl. Season with Kosar salt and freshly ground pepper allow standing for at least 30 minutes or up to 24 hours. Make 1/2 cup.
7. Make Chimichurri: Combine parsley, white wine vinegar, olive oil, garlic, jalapeño, and fresh oregano in a bowl. It is seasoned with Kosar salt. Face 2/3 glass.
8. It is served with lemon wedges, tartar sauce, mignon, chimiches, hot sauce, and malt vinegar.

NUTRITION: Calories: 221 Total fat: 4g Cholesterol: 94mg Fiber: 2g Protein: 12g Sodium: 327mg

29. Crab Chicken

Preparation Time:20 minutes
Cooking Time:40 minutes
Servings:8
INGREDIENTS:

- Canola oil for roasting
- 1c coarse corn flour
- 1/2 Cup Flour, spoon, and surface used
- 3/4 Cup Baking powder
- 1/2 spoon
- 1/4 tablespoon
- Sare Kosar
- 2 arpagic, finely chopped
- 1 tablespoon crushed peas
- Eat 8 ounces of claw crab meat (2.11 c)
- 4 oz. of Gruyère cheese, chilled (about 1 cup)
- 1 c Dough water
- 1 you tie

DIRECTIONS:

1. Heat 1 1/2-inch oil in a large Dutch oven over medium heat up to 350 degrees F (deep-fry).
2. Meanwhile, mix the cornmeal, flour, baking powder, cayenne, baking soda, and 3/4 teaspoon salt in a bowl. Add onion and onion and mix to combine. Add the crab meat and cheese and mix with a fork to combine. In the center of a well, add the butter and egg and mix to combine.
3. Spoon soup into the hot oil and be careful not to spill the pan and fry, occasionally turning until browned, 3 to 5 minutes. Transfer to a sheet of paper towel — season with salt repeat with the remaining dough.

NUTRITION: Calories: 351 Total fat: 4g Cholesterol: 94mg Fiber: 2g Protein: 12g Sodium: 319mg

30. Slow Lentil Soup

Preparation Time:10 minutes
Cooking Time:20 minutes
Servings:6
INGREDIENTS:

- 4 cups (1 quart) of low sodium vegetable juice
- 1 (14 oz.) tomatoes can (no leak)
- 1 small, fried yellow onion
- 1 medium carrot, sliced
- 1 medium-sized celery stalk, one-piece
- 1 cup green lentils
- 1 teaspoon of olive oil, plus more for cedar
- 2 cloves of garlic, turn
- 1 teaspoon Kosar salt
- 1 teaspoon tomato paste
- 1 leaf
- 1/2 teaspoon below ground
- 1/2 teaspoon of ground coriander
- 1/4 teaspoon of smoked peppers
- 2 tablespoons red wine vinegar
- Serving options: plain yogurt, olive oil, freshly chopped parsley or coriander leaves

DIRECTIONS:

1. Put all ingredients, except vinegar, in a slow cooker for 1/3 to 2-4 quarts and mix to combine. Cover and cook in the LOW settings for about 8 hours until the lentil is tender.
2. Remove bay leaf and mix in red wine vinegar. If desired, place a pot, a drop of olive oil and fresh parsley or crushed liquid in a bowl.

NUTRITION: Calories: 231 Total fat: 4g Cholesterol: 64mg Fiber: 2g Protein: 12g Sodium: 368mg

31. Light Bang Shrimp Paste

Preparation Time: 10 minutes
Cooking Time:20 minutes
Servings:4
INGREDIENTS:

- For crunchy crumbs:
- 1 tablespoon oil without butter
- Fresh cups or pancakes
- 1/8 teaspoon Kosar salt
- 1/8 teaspoon fresh black pepper
- Pepper racks
- Spend garlic powder
- For shrimp pasta:
- Cooking spray
- ½ cup of Greek yogurt whole milk
- 2 tablespoons of Asian sweet pepper sauce, such as the iconic eel
- 1 teaspoon of honey
- ¼ teaspoon of garlic powder
- The juice is divided into 2 medium lemons (about 1/4 glass)
- 12 ounces of dried spaghetti
- 1 cup shrimp without skin and peeled
- 1 teaspoon Kosar salt, plus for pasta juice
- ¼ teaspoon fresh black pepper
- 1/8 teaspoon cayenne pepper
- 2 Moderated onions, sliced, sliced

DIRECTIONS:

1. Make crisp crumbs:
2. Over a low heat, defrost the butter in a skillet. Add crumbs, salt, black pepper, cayenne pepper, and garlic powder. Cook while constantly stirring, until golden, crispy and fragrant. It will take 4 - 5 minutes, then put it aside.
3. Make shrimps:
4. Place a shelf in the middle of the oven and heat to 400 degrees Fahrenheit. Cover with a lightly cooked baking sheet with cooking spray. Put it aside
5. Boil salt water in a big pot. Meanwhile, chop yogurt, pepper sauce, honey, garlic powder and half of the lemon juice in a small bowl. Put it aside
6. Put the pasta when the water is boiling and boil the pasta for up to 10 minutes or as instructed. Dry the shrimps and place them on a sheet of ready-made cooking. Season with salt, black pepper and coffee and mix to cook. It stretches in a uniform layer. Roast once, until the shrimps are matte and pink, 6 to 8 minutes. Pour the remaining lemon juice over the shrimps and pour over it and pour the flavored pieces onto the baking sheet.
7. Evacuate the pasta and return it to the pot. Pour into the yogurt sauce and serve until well cooked. Put shrimp and juice on baking sheet with half of the onion and lightly add it again. Generously sprinkle each portion with a crunchy crumb and remaining onion. Serve immediately.

NUTRITION: Calories: 351 Total fat: 4g Cholesterol: 94mg Fiber: 2g Protein: 12g Sodium: 327mg

32. Sweet and Smoked Salmon

Preparation Time:35 minutes
Cooking Time:1 hour
Servings:8
INGREDIENTS:

- 2 tablespoons light brown sugar
- 2 tablespoons smoked peppers
- 1 tablespoon shaved lemon peel
- Sare Kosar
- Freshly chopped black pepper
- Salmon fillets on the skin 1/2 kilogram

DIRECTIONS:

1. Soak a large plate (about 15 cm by 7 inches) in water for 1 to 2 hours.
2. It is heated over medium heat. Combine sugar, pepper, lemon zest, and 1/2 teaspoon of salt and pepper in a bowl. Mix the salmon with the salt and rub the mixture of spices in all parts of the meat.
3. Put the salmon on the wet plate, skin down — oven, covered, in the desired color, 25 to 28 minutes for medium.

NUTRITION: Calories: 321 Total fat: 4g Cholesterol: 54mg Fiber: 2g Protein: 12g Sodium: 337mg

33. Chocolate Cherry Crunch Granola

Preparation Time:10 minutes
Cooking Time:20 minutes
Servings:6
INGREDIENTS:

- 3 cups rolled oats
- 2 cups assorted seeds, such as sesame, chia, sunflower, and pepitas (hulled pumpkin seeds)
- 1 cup sliced almonds
- 1 cup unsweetened coconut flakes
- 2 teaspoons vanilla extract
- 2 teaspoons ground cinnamon
- 1 teaspoon fine sea salt
- ½ cup cocoa powder
- ½ cup pure maple syrup
- ¼ cup coconut oil or canola oil
- 1 cup dried cherries (unsweetened, if possible)
- 1 cup chocolate chips

DIRECTIONS:

1. Preheat the oven to 350°F. Spread 2 large baking sheets with parchment paper.
2. In a large bowl, stir together the oats, seeds, almonds, and coconut. Add the vanilla, cinnamon, salt, and cocoa powder. Stir to combine.
3. In a fry pan over low heat, heat the maple syrup and coconut oil. Pour the warm syrup and oil over the oat mixture and stir to coat. On the prepared baking sheets, spread the granola in even layers.
4. Bake for 15 to 18 minutes, scraping and mixing occasionally, then remove from the oven.
5. Put in the dried cherries and chocolate chips, then return to the oven, now turned off but still warm, and let the granola cool and dry completely.

NUTRITION: Calories: 570 Total fat: 31g Cholesterol: 94mg Fiber: 2g Protein: 12g Sodium: 204mg

34. Creamy Raspberry Pomegranate Smoothie

Preparation Time:5 minutes
Cooking Time:5 minutes
Servings:1
INGREDIENTS:

- 1½ cups pomegranate juice
- ½ cup unsweetened coconut milk
- 1 scoop vanilla protein powder (plant-based if you need it to be dairy-free)
- 2 packed cups fresh baby spinach
- 1 cup frozen raspberries
- 1 frozen banana (see Tip)
- 1 to 2 tablespoons freshly compressed lemon juice

DIRECTIONS:

1. In a blender, combine the pomegranate juice and coconut milk. Add the protein powder and spinach. Give these a whirl to break down the spinach.
2. Add the raspberries, banana, and lemon juice, then top it off with ice. Blend until smooth and frothy.

NUTRITION: Calories: 303 Total fat: 3g Cholesterol: 0mg Fiber: 2g Protein: 15g Sodium: 165mg

35. Mango Coconut Oatmeal

Preparation Time:5 minutes
Cooking Time:5 minutes
Servings:2
INGREDIENTS:

- 1½ cups water
- ½ cup 5-minute steel cut oats
- ¼ cup unsweetened canned coconut milk, plus more for serving (optional)
- 1 tablespoon pure maple syrup
- 1 teaspoon sesame seeds
- Dash ground cinnamon
- 1 mango, stripped, pitted, and divide into slices
- 1 tablespoon unsweetened coconut flakes

DIRECTION:

1. In a fry pan over high heat, boil water. Put the oats and lower the heat. Cook, stirring occasionally, for 5 minutes.
2. Put in the coconut milk, maple syrup, and salt to combine.
3. Get two bowls and sprinkle with the sesame seeds and cinnamon. Top with sliced mango and coconut flakes.

NUTRITION: Calories: 373 Total fat: 11g Cholesterol: 0mg Fiber: 2g Protein: 12g Sodium: 167mg

36. Spiced Sweet Potato Hash with Cilantro-Lime Cream

Preparation Time:20 minutes
Cooking Time:30 minutes
Servings:2
INGREDIENTS:

- For the cilantro-lime cream
- 1 avocado, halved and pitted
- ¼ cup packed fresh cilantro leaves and stems
- 2 tablespoons freshly squeezed lime juice
- 1 garlic clove, peeled
- 1 teaspoon kosher salt
- ½ teaspoon ground cumin
- 2 tablespoons extra-virgin olive oil
- For the hash
- ½ teaspoon kosher salt
- 1 large sweet potato, cut into ¾-inch pieces
- 2 tablespoons extra-virgin olive oil
- 1 onion, thinly sliced
- 2 garlic cloves, crushed
- 1 red bell pepper, thinly sliced
- 1 teaspoon ground cumin
- ¼ teaspoon ground turmeric
- Pinch freshly ground black pepper
- 2 tablespoons fresh cilantro leaves, chopped
- ½ jalapeño pepper, seeded and chopped (optional)
- Hot sauce, for serving (optional)

DIRECTIONS:

1. To make the cilantro-lime cream
2. Add the avocado flesh in a food compressor Add the cilantro, lime juice, garlic, salt, and cumin. Whirl until smooth. When the processor is running slowly, softly. Taste and adjust seasonings, as needed. If you do not have a food processor or blender, simply mash the avocado well with a fork; the results will have more texture, but will still work. Cover and refrigerate until ready to serve.
3. To make the hash
4. Boil a salt water in a medium pot over high heat. Add the sweet potato and cook for about 20 minutes until tender. Drain thoroughly.
5. Heat olive oil in a big skillet over low heat until it shimmers. Add the onion and sauté for about 4 minutes until translucent. Put the garlic and cook, turning, for about 30 seconds. Add the cooked sweet potato and red bell pepper. Season the hash with cumin, salt, turmeric, and pepper. For 5 to 7 minutes, Saute until the sweet potatoes are golden and the red bell pepper is soft.
6. Divide the sweet potatoes between 2 bowls and spoon the sauce over them. Scatter the cilantro and jalapeño (if using) over each and serve with hot sauce (if using).

NUTRITION: Calories: 520 Total fat: 43g Cholesterol: 0mg Fiber: 2g Protein: 12g Sodium: 1719mg

37. Open-Face Egg Sandwiches with Cilantro-Jalapeño Spread

Preparation Time:20 minutes
Cooking Time:10 minutes
Servings:2
INGREDIENTS:

- For the cilantro and jalapeño spread
- 1 cup filled up fresh cilantro leaves and stems (about 1 bunch)
- 1 jalapeño pepper, seeded, and roughly chopped
- ½ cup extra-virgin olive oil
- ¼ cup pepitas (hulled pumpkin seeds), raw or roasted
- 2 garlic cloves, thinly sliced
- 1 tablespoon freshly squeezed lime juice
- 1 teaspoon kosher salt
- For the eggs
- 4 large eggs
- ¼ cup milk
- ¼ to ½ teaspoon kosher salt
- 2 tablespoons butter
- For the sandwich
- 2 slices bread
- 1 tablespoon butter
- 1 avocado, halved, pitted and divided into slices
- Microgreens or sprouts, for garnish

DIRECTIONS:

1. To make the cilantro and jalapeño spread
2. In a food processor, combine the cilantro, jalapeño, oil, pepitas, garlic, lime juice, and salt. Whirl until smooth. Refrigerate if making in advance; otherwise set aside.
3. To make the eggs
4. In a medium bowl, whisk the eggs, milk, and salt.
5. Dissolve the butter in a skillet over low heat, swirling to coat the bottom of the pan. Pour in the whisked eggs. Cook until they begin to set then, using a heatproof spatula, push them to the sides, allowing the uncooked portions to run into the bottom of the skillet. Continue until the eggs are set.
6. To assemble the sandwiches
7. Toast the bed and spread with butter.
8. Spread a spoonful of the cilantro-jalapeño spread on each piece of toast. Top each with scrambled eggs.
9. Arrange avocado over each sandwich and garnish with microgreens.

NUTRITION: Calories: 711 Total fat: 4g Cholesterol: 54mg Fiber: 12g Protein: 12g Sodium: 327mg

38. Scrambled Eggs with Soy Sauce and Broccoli Slaw

Preparation Time:5 minutes
Cooking Time:10 minutes
Servings: 2
INGREDIENTS:

- 1 tablespoon peanut oil, divided
- 4 large eggs
- ½ to 1 tablespoon soy sauce, tamari, or Bragg's liquid aminos
- 1 tablespoon water
- 1 cup shredded broccoli slaw or other shredded vegetable
- Kosher salt
- Chopped fresh cilantro, for serving
- Hot sauce, for serving

DIRECTIONS:

1. In a medium nonstick skillet or cast-iron skillet over medium heat, heat 2 teaspoons of peanut oil, swirling to coat the skillet.
2. In a small bowl, whip the eggs, soy sauce, and water until smooth. Pour the eggs into the pan and let the bottom set. Using a wooden spoon, spread the eggs from one side to the other a couple times so the uncooked portions on top pool into the bottom. Cook until the eggs are set.
3. In a medium container, stir together the broccoli slaw, remaining 1 teaspoon of peanut oil, and a touch of salt. Divide the slaw between 2 plates.
4. Top with the eggs and scatter cilantro on each serving. Serve with hot sauce.

NUTRITION: Calories: 222 Total fat: 4g Cholesterol: 374mg Fiber: 2g Protein: 12g Sodium: 737mg

39. Tasty Breakfast Donuts

Preparation Time: 5 minutes
Cooking Time: 5 minutes
Servings: 4
INGREDIENTS:

- 43 grams' cream cheese
- 2 eggs
- 2 tablespoons almond flour
- 2 tablespoons erythritol
- 1 ½ tablespoons coconut flour
- ½ teaspoon baking powder
- ½ teaspoon vanilla extract
- 5 drops Stevia (liquid form)
- 2 strips bacon, fried until crispy

DIRECTIONS:

1. Rub coconut oil over donut maker and turn on.
2. Pulse all ingredients except bacon in a blender or food processor until smooth (should take around 1 minute).
3. Pour batter into donut maker, leaving 1/10 in each round for rising.
4. Leave for 3 minutes before flipping each donut. Leave for another 2 minutes or until fork comes out clean when piercing them.
5. Take donuts out and let cool.
6. Repeat steps 1-5 until all batter is used.
7. Crumble bacon into bits and use to top donuts.

NUTRITION: Calories: 60 Fat: 5g Carbs: 1g Fiber: 0g Protein: 3g

40. Cheesy Spicy Bacon Bowls

Preparation Time: 10 minutes
Cooking Time: 22 minutes
Servings: 12
INGREDIENTS:

- 6 strips Bacon, pan fried until cooked but still malleable
- 4 eggs
- 60 grams' cheddar cheese
- 40 grams' cream cheese, grated
- 2 Jalapenos, sliced and seeds removed
- 2 tablespoons coconut oil
- ¼ teaspoon onion powder
- ¼ teaspoon garlic powder
- Dash of salt and pepper

DIRECTIONS:

1. Preheat oven to 375 degrees Fahrenheit
2. In a bowl, beat together eggs, cream cheese, jalapenos (minus 6 slices), coconut oil, onion powder, garlic powder, and salt and pepper.
3. Using leftover bacon grease on a muffin tray, rubbing it into each insert. Place bacon wrapped inside the parameters of each insert.
4. Pour beaten mixture half way up each bacon bowl.
5. Garnish each bacon bowl with cheese and leftover jalapeno slices (placing one on top of each).
6. Leave in the oven for about 22 minutes, or until egg is thoroughly cooked and cheese is bubbly.
7. Remove from oven and let cool until edible.
8. Enjoy!

NUTRITION: Calories: 259 Fat: 24g Carbs: 1g Fiber: 0g Protein: 10g

41. Goat Cheese Zucchini Kale Quiche

Preparation Time: 35 minutes
Cooking Time: 1 hour 10 minutes
Servings: 4
INGREDIENTS:

- 4 large eggs
- 8 ounces' fresh zucchini, sliced
- 10 ounces' kale
- 3 garlic cloves (minced)
- 1 cup soy milk
- 1 ounce's goat cheese
- 1cup grated parmesan
- 1cup shredded cheddar cheese
- 2 teaspoons olive oil
- Salt & pepper, to taste

DIRECTIONS:

1. Preheat oven to 350°F.
2. Heat 1 tsp of olive oil in a saucepan over medium-high heat. Sauté garlic for 1 minute until flavored.
3. Add the zucchini and cook for another 5-7 minutes until soft.
4. Beat the eggs and then add a little milk and Parmesan cheese.
5. Meanwhile, heat the remaining olive oil in another saucepan and add the cabbage. Cover and cook for 5 minutes until dry.
6. Slightly grease a baking dish with cooking spray and spread the kale leaves across the bottom. Add the zucchini and top with goat cheese.
7. Pour the egg, milk and parmesan mixture evenly over the other ingredients. Top with cheddar cheese.
8. Bake for 50–60 minutes until golden brown. Check the center of the quiche, it should have a solid consistency.
9. Let chill for a few minutes before serving.

NUTRITION: Total Carbohydrates: 15g Dietary Fiber: 2g Net Carbs: 13g Protein: 19g Total Fat: 18g Calories: 290

42. Cream Cheese Egg Breakfast

Preparation Time: 5 minutes
Cooking Time: 5 minutes
Servings: 4
INGREDIENTS:

- 2 eggs, beaten
- 1 tablespoon butter
- 2 tablespoons soft cream cheese with chives

DIRECTIONS:

1. Melt the butter in a small skillet. Add the eggs and cream cheese. Stir and cook to desired doneness.

NUTRITION: Calories: 341 Fat: 31g Protein: 15g Carbohydrate: 0g Dietary Fiber: 3g

43. Avocado Red Peppers Roasted Scrambled Eggs

Preparation Time: 10 minutes
Cooking Time: 12 minutes
Servings: 3
INGREDIENTS:

- 1/2 tablespoon butter
- Eggs, 2
- 1/2 roasted red pepper, about 1 1/2 ounces
- 1/2 small avocado, coarsely chopped, about 2 1/4 ounces
- Salt, to taste

DIRECTIONS:

1. In a nonstick skillet, heat the butter over medium heat. Break the eggs into the pan and break the yolks with a spoon. sprinkle with a little salt.
2. Stir to stir and continue stirring until the eggs start to come out. Quickly add the bell peppers and avocado.
3. Cook and stir until the eggs suit your taste. Adjust the seasoning, if necessary.

NUTRITION: Calories: 317 Fat: 26g Protein: 14g Dietary Fiber: 5g Net Carbs: 4g

44. Mushroom Quickie Scramble

Preparation Time: 10 minutes
Cooking Time: 10 minutes
Servings: 4
INGREDIENTS:

- 3 small sized eggs, whisked
- 4 pcs. bella mushrooms
- ½ cup of spinach
- ¼ cup of red bell peppers
- 2 deli ham slices
- 1 tablespoon of ghee or coconut oil
- Salt & pepper to taste

DIRECTIONS:

1. Chop the ham and veggies.
2. Put half a tbsp of butter in a frying pan and heat until melted.
3. Sauté the ham and vegetables in a frying pan then set aside.
4. Get a new frying pan and heat the remaining butter.
5. Add the whisked eggs into the second pan while stirring continuously to avoid overcooking.
6. When the eggs are done, sprinkle with salt & pepper to taste.
7. Add the ham and veggies to the pan with the eggs.
8. Mix well.
9. Remove from burner and transfer to a plate.
10. Serve and enjoy.

NUTRITION: Calories: 350 Total Fat: 29 g Protein: 21 g Total Carbs: 5 g

45. Coconut Coffee and Ghee

Preparation Time: 10 minutes
Cooking Time: 10 minutes
Servings: 5
INGREDIENTS:

- ½ Tbsp. of coconut oil
- ½ Tbsp. of ghee
- 1 to 2 cups of preferred coffee (or rooibos or black tea, if preferred)
- 1 Tbsp. of coconut or almond milk

DIRECTIONS:

1. Place the almond (or coconut) milk, coconut oil, ghee and coffee in a blender (or milk frothier).
2. mix for around 10 seconds or until the coffee turns creamy and foamy.
3. Pour contents into a coffee cup.
4. Serve immediately and enjoy.

NUTRITION: Calories: 150 Total Fat: 15 g Protein: 0 g Total Carbs: 0 g Net Carbs: 0 g

46. Yummy Veggie Waffles

Preparation Time: 10 minutes
Cooking Time: 9 minutes
Servings: 3
INGREDIENTS:

- 3 cups raw cauliflower, grated
- 1 cup cheddar cheese
- 1 cup mozzarella cheese
- ½ cup parmesan
- 1/3 cup chives, finely sliced
- 6 eggs
- 1 teaspoon garlic powder
- 1 teaspoon onion powder
- ½ teaspoon chili flakes
- Dash of salt and pepper

DIRECTIONS:

1. Turn waffle maker on.
2. In a bowl mix all the listed ingredients very well until incorporated.
3. Once waffle maker is hot, distribute waffle mixture into the insert.
4. Let cook for about 9 minutes, flipping at 6 minutes.
5. Remove from waffle maker and set aside.
6. Repeat the previous steps with the rest of the batter until gone (should come out to 4 waffles)
7. Serve and enjoy!

NUTRITION: Calories: 390 Fat: 28g Carbs: 6g Fiber: 2g Protein: 30g

47. Omega 3 Breakfast Shake

Preparation Time: 5 minutes
Cooking Time: 5 minutes
Servings: 2
INGREDIENTS:

- 1 cup vanilla almond milk (unsweetened)
- 2 tablespoons blueberries
- 1 ½ tablespoons flaxseed meal
- 1 tablespoon MCT Oil
- ¾ tablespoon banana extract
- ½ tablespoon chia seeds
- 5 drops Stevia (liquid form)
- 1/8 tablespoon Xanthan gum

DIRECTIONS:

1. In a blender, pulse vanilla almond milk, banana extract, Stevia, and 3 ice cubes.
2. When smooth, add blueberries and pulse.
3. Once blueberries are thoroughly incorporated, add flaxseed meal and chia seeds.
4. Let sit for 5 minutes.
5. After 5 minutes, pulse again until all ingredients are nicely distributed. Serve and enjoy

NUTRITION: Calories: 264 Fats: 25g Carbs: 7g Protein: 4g

48. Bacon Spaghetti Squash Carbonara

Preparation Time: 20 minutes
Cooking Time: 40 minutes
Servings: 4
INGREDIENTS:

- 1 small spaghetti squash
- 6 ounces' bacon (roughly chopped)
- 1 large tomato (sliced)
- 2 chives (chopped)
- 1 garlic clove (minced)
- 6 ounces' low-fat cottage cheese
- 1 cup Gouda cheese (grated)
- 2 tablespoons olive oil
- Salt and pepper, to taste

DIRECTIONS:

1. Preheat the oven to 350°F.
2. Cut the squash spaghetti in half, brush with some olive oil and bake for 20–30 minutes, skin side up. Remove from the oven and remove the core with a fork, creating the spaghetti.
3. Heat one tablespoon of olive oil in a skillet. Cook the bacon for about 1 minute until crispy.
4. Quickly wipe out the pan with paper towels.
5. Heat another tablespoon of oil and sauté the garlic, tomato and chives for 2–3 minutes. Add the spaghetti and sauté for another 5 minutes, stirring occasionally to keep from burning.
6. Begin to add the cottage cheese, about 2 tablespoons at a time. If the sauce becomes thicken, add about a cup of water. The sauce should be creamy, but not too runny or thick. Allow to cook for another 3 minutes.
7. Serve immediately.

NUTRITION: Calories: 305 Total Fat: 21g Net Carbs: 8g Protein: 18g

49. Lime Bacon Thyme Muffins

Preparation Time: 10 minutes
Cooking Time: 20 minutes
Servings: 3
INGREDIENTS:

- 3 cups of almond flour
- 4 medium-sized eggs
- 1 cup of bacon bits
- 2 tsp. of lemon thyme
- ½ cup of melted ghee
- 1 tsp. of baking soda
- ½ tsp. of salt, to taste

DIRECTIONS:

1. Pre-heat oven to 350° F.
2. Put ghee in mixing bowl and melt.
3. Add baking soda and almond flour.
4. Put the eggs in.
5. Add the lemon thyme (if preferred, other herbs or spices may be used).
6. Drizzle with salt.
7. Mix all ingredients well.
8. Sprinkle with bacon bits
9. Line the muffin pan with liners.
10. Spoon mixture into the pan, filling the pan to about ¾ full.
11. Bake for about 20 minutes. Test by inserting a toothpick into a muffin. If it comes out clean, then the muffins are done.
12. Serve immediately.

NUTRITION: Calories: 300 Total Fat: 28 g Protein: 11 g Total Carbs: 6 g Fiber: 3 g

50. Gluten -Free Pancakes

Preparation Time: 5 minutes
Cooking Time: 2 minutes
Servings: 2
INGREDIENTS:

- 6 eggs
- 1 cup low-fat cream cheese
- 1 1/12; teaspoons baking powder
- 1 scoop protein powder
- 1/4; cup almond meal
- ¼ teaspoon salt

DIRECTIONS:

1. Combine dry ingredients in a food processor. Add the eggs one after another and then the cream cheese. Edit until you have a blast.
2. Lightly grease a skillet with cooking spray and place over medium-high heat.
3. Pour the batter into the pan. Turn the pan gently to create round pancakes.
4. Cook for about 2 minutes on each side.
5. Serve pancakes with your favorite topping.

NUTRITION: Dietary Fiber: 1g Net Carbs: 5g Protein: 25g Total Fat: 14g Calories: 288

51. Mushroom & Spinach Omelet

Preparation Time: 20 minutes
Cooking Time: 20 minutes
Servings: 3
INGREDIENTS:

- 2 tablespoons butter, divided
- 6-8 fresh mushrooms, sliced, 5 ounces
- Chives, chopped, optional
- Salt and pepper, to taste
- 1 handful baby spinach, about 1/2 ounce
- Pinch garlic powder
- 4 eggs, beaten
- 1-ounce shredded Swiss cheese,

DIRECTIONS:

1. In a very large saucepan, sauté the mushrooms in 1 tablespoon of butter until soft. season with salt, pepper and garlic.
2. Remove the mushrooms from the pan and keep warm. Heat the remaining tablespoon of butter in the same skillet over medium heat.
3. Beat the eggs with a little salt and pepper and add to the hot butter. Turn the pan over to coat the entire bottom of the pan with egg. Once the egg is almost out, place the cheese over the middle of the tortilla.
4. Fill the cheese with spinach leaves and hot mushrooms. Let cook for about a minute for the spinach to start to wilt. Fold the empty side of the tortilla carefully over the filling and slide it onto a plate and sprinkle with chives, if desired.
5. Alternatively, you can make two tortillas using half the mushroom, spinach, and cheese filling in each.

NUTRITION: Calories: 321 Fat: 26g Protein: 19g Carbohydrate: 4g Dietary Fiber: 1g

MAINS

52. Balsamic Beef and Mushrooms Mix

Preparation Time: 5 minutes
Cooking Time: 8 hours
Servings: 4
INGREDIENTS:

- 2 pounds' beef, cut into strips
- ¼ cup balsamic vinegar
- 2 cups beef stock
- 1 tablespoon ginger, grated
- Juice of ½ lemon
- 1 cup brown mushrooms, sliced
- A pinch of salt and black pepper
- 1 teaspoon ground cinnamon

DIRECTIONS:

1. In your slow cooker, mix all the ingredients, cover and cook on low for 8 hours.
2. Divide everything between plates and serve.

NUTRITION: Calories: 446 Fat: 14g Fiber: 0.6g Carbs: 2.9 g Protein: 70g

53. Oregano Pork Mix

Preparation Time: 5 minutes
Cooking Time: 7 hours and 6 minutes
Servings: 4
INGREDIENTS:

- 2 pounds' pork roast
- 7 ounces' tomato paste
- 1 yellow onion, chopped
- 1 cup beef stock
- 2 tablespoons ground cumin
- 2 tablespoons olive oil
- 2 tablespoons fresh oregano, chopped
- 1 tablespoon garlic, minced
- ½ cup fresh thyme, chopped

DIRECTIONS:

1. Heat up a sauté pan with the oil over medium-high heat, add the roast, brown it for 3 minutes on both side and then transfer to your slow cooker.
2. Add the remaining ingredients, toss a bit, cover and cook on low for 7 hours.
3. Slice the roast, divide it between plates and serve.

NUTRITION: Calories: 623 Fat: 30.1g Fiber: 6.2g Carbs: 19.3g Protein: 69.2g

54. Simple Beef Roast

Preparation Time: 10 minutes
Cooking Time: 8 hours
Servings: 8
INGREDIENTS:

- 5 pounds' beef roast
- 2 tablespoons Italian seasoning
- 1 cup beef stock
- 1 tablespoon sweet paprika
- 3 tablespoons olive oil

DIRECTIONS:

1. In your slow cooker, mix all the ingredients, cover and cook on low for 8 hours.
2. Carve the roast, divide it between plates and serve.

NUTRITION: Calories: 587 Fat: 24.1g Fiber: 0.3g Carbs: 0.9g Protein: 86.5g

55. Chicken Breast Soup

Preparation Time: 5 minutes
Cooking Time: 4 hours
Servings: 4
INGREDIENTS:

- 3 chicken breasts, skinless, boneless, cubed
- 2 celery stalks, chopped
- 2 carrots, chopped
- 2 tablespoons olive oil
- 1 red onion, chopped
- 3 garlic cloves, minced
- 4 cups chicken stock
- 1 tablespoon parsley, chopped

DIRECTIONS:

1. In your slow cooker, mix all the ingredients except the parsley, cover and cook on High for 4 hours.
2. Add the parsley, stir, ladle the soup into bowls and serve.

NUTRITION: Calories: 445 Fat: 21.1g Fiber: 1.6g Carbs: 7.4g Protein: 54.3g

56. Cauliflower Curry

Preparation Time: 5 minutes
Cooking Time: 5 hours
Servings: 4
INGREDIENTS:

- 1 cauliflower head, florets separated
- 2 carrots, sliced
- 1 red onion, chopped
- ¾ cup coconut milk
- 2 garlic cloves, minced
- 2 tablespoons curry powder
- A pinch of salt and black pepper
- 1 tablespoon red pepper flakes
- 1 teaspoon garam masala

DIRECTIONS:

1. In your slow cooker, mix all the ingredients.
2. Cover, cook on high for 5 hours, divide into bowls and serve.

NUTRITION: Calories: 160 Fat: 11.5g Fiber: 5.4g Carbs: 14.7g Protein: 3.6g

57. Pork and Peppers Chili

Preparation Time: 5 minutes
Cooking Time: 8 hours and 5 minutes
Servings: 4
INGREDIENTS:

- 1 red onion, chopped
- 2 pounds' pork, ground
- 4 garlic cloves, minced
- 2 red bell peppers, chopped
- 1 celery stalk, chopped
- 25 ounces' fresh tomatoes, peeled, crushed
- ¼ cup green chilies, chopped
- 2 tablespoons fresh oregano, chopped
- 2 tablespoons chili powder
- A pinch of salt and black pepper
- A drizzle of olive oil

DIRECTIONS:

1. Heat up a sauté pan with the oil over medium-high heat and add the onion, garlic and the meat. Mix and brown for 5 minutes then transfer to your slow cooker.
2. Add the rest of the ingredients, toss, cover and cook on low for 8 hours.
3. Divide everything into bowls and serve.

NUTRITION: Calories: 448 Fat: 13g Fiber: 6.6g Carbs: 20.2g Protein: 63g

58. Greek Style Quesadillas

Preparation Time: 10 minutes
Cooking Time: 10 minutes
Servings: 4
INGREDIENTS:

- 4 whole wheat tortillas
- 1 cup Mozzarella cheese, shredded
- 1 cup fresh spinach, chopped
- 2 tablespoon Greek yogurt
- 1 egg, beaten
- ¼ cup green olives, sliced
- 1 tablespoon olive oil
- 1/3 cup fresh cilantro, chopped

DIRECTIONS:

1. In the bowl, combine together Mozzarella cheese, spinach, yogurt, egg, olives, and cilantro.
2. Then pour olive oil in the skillet.
3. In the skillet Place one tortilla and spread it with Mozzarella mixture.
4. Top it with the second tortilla and spread it with cheese mixture again.
5. Then place the third tortilla and spread it with all remaining cheese mixture.
6. Cover it with the last tortilla and fry it for 5 minutes from each side over the medium heat.

NUTRITION: Calories: 193 Fat: 7.7g Fiber: 3.2g Carbs: 23.6g Protein: 8.3g

59. Light Paprika Moussaka

Preparation Time: 15 minutes
Cooking Time: 45 minutes
Servings: 3
INGREDIENTS:

- 1 eggplant, trimmed
- 1 cup ground chicken
- 1/3 cup white onion, diced
- 3 oz. Cheddar cheese, shredded
- 1 potato, sliced
- 1 teaspoon olive oil
- 1 teaspoon salt
- ½ cup milk
- 1 tablespoon butter
- 1 tablespoon ground paprika
- 1 tablespoon Italian seasoning
- 1 teaspoon tomato paste

DIRECTIONS:

1. Slice the eggplant in length and sprinkle with salt.
2. In the skillet Pour olive oil and add sliced potato.
3. Roast potato for 2 minutes from each side.
4. Then transfer it in the plate.
5. Put eggplant in the skillet and roast it for 2 minutes from each side too.
6. In the pan Pour milk and bring it to boil.
7. Add tomato paste, Italian seasoning, paprika, butter, and Cheddar cheese.
8. Then mix up together onion with ground chicken.
9. Arrange the sliced potato in the casserole in one layer.
10. Then add ½ part of all sliced eggplants.
11. Spread the eggplants with ½ part of chicken mixture.
12. Then add remaining eggplants.
13. Pour the milk mixture over the eggplants.
14. Bake moussaka for 30 minutes at 355F.

NUTRITION: Calories: 387 Fat: 21.2g Fiber: 8.9g Carbs: 26.3g Protein: 25.4g

60. Cucumber Bowl with Spices and Greek Yogurt

Preparation Time: 10 minutes
Cooking Time: 20 minutes
Servings: 3
INGREDIENTS:

- 4 cucumbers
- ½ teaspoon chili pepper
- ¼ cup fresh parsley, chopped
- ¾ cup fresh dill, chopped
- 2 tablespoons lemon juice
- ½ teaspoon salt
- ½ teaspoon ground black pepper
- ¼ teaspoon sage
- ½ teaspoon dried oregano
- 1/3 cup Greek yogurt

DIRECTIONS:

1. Make the cucumber dressing: blend the dill and parsley until you get green mash.
2. Then combine together green mash with lemon juice, salt, ground black pepper, sage, dried oregano, Greek yogurt, and chili pepper.
3. Churn the mixture well.
4. Chop the cucumbers roughly and combine them with cucumber dressing. Mix up well.
5. Refrigerate the cucumber for 20 minutes.

NUTRITION: Calories: 114 Fat: 1.6g Fiber: 4.1g Carbs: 23.2g Protein: 7.6g

61. Stuffed Bell Peppers with Quinoa

Preparation Time: 10 minutes
Cooking Time: 35 minutes
Servings: 2
INGREDIENTS:

- 2 bell peppers
- 1/3 cup quinoa
- 3 oz. chicken stock
- ¼ cup onion, diced
- ½ teaspoon salt
- ¼ teaspoon tomato paste
- ½ teaspoon dried oregano
- 1/3 cup sour cream
- 1 teaspoon paprika

DIRECTIONS:

1. Trim the peppers and remove the seeds.
2. Then combine together chicken stock and quinoa in the pan.
3. Add salt and boil the ingredients for 10 minutes or until quinoa will soak all liquid.
4. Then combine together cooked quinoa with dried oregano, tomato paste, and onion.
5. Fill the bell peppers with the quinoa mixture and arrange in the casserole mold.
6. Add sour cream and bake the peppers for 25 minutes at 365F.
7. Serve the cooked peppers with sour cream sauce from the casserole mold.

NUTRITION: Calories: 237 Fat: 10.3 Fiber: 4.5 Carbs: 31.3 Protein: 6.9

62. Mediterranean Burrito

Preparation Time: 10 minutes
Cooking Time: 0 minutes
Servings: 2
INGREDIENTS:

- 2 wheat tortillas
- 2 oz. red kidney beans, canned, drained
- 2 tablespoons hummus
- 2 teaspoons tahini sauce
- 1 cucumber
- 2 lettuce leaves
- 1 tablespoon lime juice
- 1 teaspoon olive oil
- ½ teaspoon dried oregano

DIRECTIONS:

1. Mash the red kidney beans until you get a puree.
2. Then spread the wheat tortillas with beans mash from one side.
3. Add hummus and tahini sauce.
4. Cut the cucumber into the wedges and place them over tahini sauce.
5. Then add lettuce leaves.
6. Make the dressing: mix up together olive oil, dried oregano, and lime juice.
7. Drizzle the lettuce leaves with the dressing and wrap the wheat tortillas in the shape of burritos.

NUTRITION: Calories: 288 Fat: 10.2 Fiber: 14.6 Carbs: 38.2 Protein: 12.5

63. Sweet Potato Bacon Mash

Preparation Time: 10 minutes
Cooking Time: 20 minutes
Servings: 4
INGREDIENTS:

- 3 sweet potatoes, peeled
- 4 oz. bacon, chopped
- 1 cup chicken stock
- 1 tablespoon butter
- 1 teaspoon salt
- 2 oz. Parmesan, grated

DIRECTIONS:

1. Dice sweet potato and put it in the pan.
2. Add chicken stock and close the lid.
3. Boil the vegetables for until they are soft.
4. After this, drain the chicken stock.
5. Mash the sweet potato with the help of the potato masher. Add grated cheese and butter.
6. Mix up together salt and chopped bacon. Fry the mixture until it is crunchy (10-15 minutes).
7. Add cooked bacon in the mashed sweet potato and mix up with the help of the spoon.
8. It is recommended to serve the meal warm or hot.

NUTRITION: Calories: 304 Fat: 18.1 Fiber: 2.9 Carbs: 18.8 Protein: 17

64. Prosciutto Wrapped Mozzarella Balls

Preparation Time: 10 minutes
Cooking Time: 10 minutes
Servings: 4
INGREDIENTS:

- 8 Mozzarella balls, cherry size
- 4 oz. bacon, sliced
- ¼ teaspoon ground black pepper
- ¾ teaspoon dried rosemary
- 1 teaspoon butter

DIRECTIONS:

1. Sprinkle the sliced bacon with ground black pepper and dried rosemary.
2. Wrap every Mozzarella ball in the sliced bacon and secure them with toothpicks.
3. Melt butter.
4. Brush wrapped Mozzarella balls with butter.
5. Line the baking tray with the parchment and arrange Mozzarella balls in it.
6. Bake the meal for 10 minutes at 365F.

NUTRITION: Calories: 323 Fat: 26.8 Fiber: 0.1 Carbs: 0.6 Protein: 20.6

65. Garlic Chicken Balls

Preparation Time: 15 minutes
Cooking Time: 10 minutes
Servings: 4
INGREDIENTS:

- 2 cups ground chicken
- 1 teaspoon minced garlic
- 1 teaspoon dried dill
- 1/3 carrot, grated
- 1 egg, beaten
- 1 tablespoon olive oil
- ¼ cup coconut flakes
- ½ teaspoon salt

DIRECTIONS:

1. In the mixing bowl mix up together ground chicken, minced garlic, dried dill, carrot, egg, and salt.
2. Stir the chicken mixture with the help of the fingertips until homogenous.
3. Then make medium balls from the mixture.
4. Coat every chicken ball in coconut flakes.
5. Heat up olive oil in the skillet.
6. Add chicken balls and cook them for 3 minutes from each side. The cooked chicken balls will have a golden-brown color.

NUTRITION: Calories: 200 Fat: 11.5 Fiber: 0.6 Carbs: 1.7 Protein: 21.9

66. Lettuce Salad with Beef Strips

Preparation Time: 10 minutes
Cooking Time: 12 minutes
Servings: 5
INGREDIENTS:

- 2 cup lettuce
- 10 oz. beef brisket
- 2 tablespoon sesame oil
- 1 tablespoon sunflower seeds
- 1 cucumber
- 1 teaspoon ground black pepper
- 1 teaspoon paprika
- 1 teaspoon Italian spices
- 2 teaspoon butter
- 1 teaspoon dried dill
- 2 tablespoon coconut milk

DIRECTIONS:

1. Cut the beef brisket into strips.
2. Sprinkle the beef strips with the ground black pepper, paprika, and dried dill.
3. Preheat the air fryer to 365 F.
4. Put the butter in the air fryer basket tray and melt it.
5. Then add the beef strips and cook them for 6 minutes on each side.
6. Meanwhile, tear the lettuce and toss it in a big salad bowl.
7. Crush the sunflower seeds and sprinkle over the lettuce.
8. Chop the cucumber into the small cubes and add to the salad bowl.
9. Then combine the sesame oil and Italian spices together. Stir the oil.
10. Combine the lettuce mixture with the coconut milk and stir it using 2 wooden spatulas.
11. When the meat is cooked – let it chill to room temperature.
12. Add the beef strips to the salad bowl.
13. Stir it gently and sprinkle the salad with the sesame oil dressing.
14. Serve the dish immediately.

NUTRITION: Calories: 199 Fat: 12.4g Carbs: 3.9g Protein: 18.1g

67. Cayenne Rib Eye Steak

Preparation Time: 10 minutes
Cooking Time: 13 minutes
Servings: 2
INGREDIENTS:

- 1-pound rib eye steak
- 1 teaspoon salt
- 1 teaspoon cayenne pepper
- ½ teaspoon chili flakes
- 3 tablespoon cream
- 1 teaspoon olive oil
- 1 teaspoon lemongrass
- 1 tablespoon butter
- 1 teaspoon garlic powder

DIRECTIONS:

1. Preheat the air fryer to 360 F.
2. Take a shallow bowl and combine the cayenne pepper, salt, chili flakes, lemongrass, and garlic powder together.
3. Mix the spices gently.
4. Sprinkle the rib eye steak with the spice mixture.
5. Melt the butter and combine it with cream and olive oil.
6. Churn the mixture.
7. Pour the churned mixture into the air fryer basket tray.
8. Add the rib eye steak.
9. Cook the steak for 13 minutes. Do not stir the steak during the cooking.
10. When the steak is cooked transfer it to a paper towel to soak all the excess fat.
11. Serve the steak. You can slice the steak if desired.

NUTRITION: Calories: 708 Fat: 59g Carbs: 2.3g Protein: 40.4g

68. Beef-Chicken Meatball Casserole

Preparation Time: 15 minutes
Cooking Time: 21 minutes
Servings: 7
INGREDIENTS:

- 1 eggplant
- 10 oz. ground chicken
- 8 oz. ground beef
- 1 teaspoon minced garlic
- 1 teaspoon ground white pepper
- 1 tomato
- 1 egg
- 1 tablespoon coconut flour
- 8 oz. Parmesan, shredded
- 2 tablespoon butter
- 1/3 cup cream

DIRECTIONS:

1. Combine the ground chicken and ground beef in a large bowl.
2. Add the minced garlic and ground white pepper.
3. In the bowl Crack the egg with the ground meat mixture and stir it carefully until well combined.
4. Then add the coconut flour and mix.
5. Make small meatballs from the ground meat.
6. Preheat the air fryer to 360 F.
7. Sprinkle the air fryer basket tray with the butter and pour the cream.
8. Peel the eggplant and chop it.
9. Put the meatballs over the cream and sprinkle them with the chopped eggplant.
10. Slice the tomato and place it over the eggplant.
11. Make a layer of shredded cheese over the sliced tomato.
12. Put the casserole in the air fryer and cook it for 21 minutes.
13. Let the casserole cool to room temperature before serving.

NUTRITION: Calories: 314 Fat: 16.8g Carbs: 7.5g Protein: 33.9g

69. Juicy Pork Chops

Preparation Time: 10 minutes
Cooking Time: 11 minutes
Servings: 3
INGREDIENTS:

- 1 teaspoon peppercorns
- 1 teaspoon kosher salt
- 1 teaspoon minced garlic
- ½ teaspoon dried rosemary
- 1 tablespoon butter
- 13 oz. pork chops

DIRECTIONS:

1. Rub the pork chops with the dried rosemary, minced garlic, and kosher salt.
2. Preheat the air fryer to 365 F.
3. Put the butter and peppercorns in the air fryer basket tray. Melt the butter.
4. Place the pork chops in the melted butter.
5. Cook the pork chops for 6 minutes.
6. Turn the pork chops over.
7. Cook the pork chops for 5 minutes more.
8. When the meat is cooked dry gently with the paper towel.
9. Serve the juicy pork chops immediately.

NUTRITION: Calories: 431, Fat: 34.4g Carbs: 0.9g Protein: 27.8

70. Chicken Goulash

Preparation Time: 10 minutes
Cooking Time: 17 minutes
Servings: 6
INGREDIENTS:

- 4 oz. chive stems
- 2 green peppers, chopped
- 1 teaspoon olive oil
- 14 oz. ground chicken
- 2 tomatoes
- ½ cup chicken stock
- 2 garlic cloves, sliced
- 1 teaspoon salt
- 1 teaspoon ground black pepper
- 1 teaspoon mustard

DIRECTIONS:

1. Chop chives roughly.
2. Spray the air fryer basket tray with the olive oil.
3. Preheat the air fryer to 365 F.
4. Put the chopped chives in the air fryer basket tray.
5. Add the chopped green pepper and cook the vegetables for 5 minutes.
6. Add the ground chicken.
7. Chop the tomatoes into the small cubes and add them in the air fryer mixture too.
8. Cook the mixture for 6 minutes more.
9. Add the chicken stock, sliced garlic cloves, salt, ground black pepper, and mustard.
10. Mix well to combine.
11. Cook the goulash for 6 minutes more.

NUTRITION: Calories: 161 Fat: 6.1g Carbs: 6g Protein: 20.3g

71. Chicken & Turkey Meatloaf

Preparation Time: 15 minutes
Cooking Time: 25 minutes
Servings: 12
INGREDIENTS:

- 3 tablespoon butter
- 10 oz. ground turkey
- 7 oz. ground chicken
- 1 teaspoon dried dill
- ½ teaspoon ground coriander
- 2 tablespoons almond flour
- 1 tablespoon minced garlic
- 3 oz. fresh spinach
- 1 teaspoon salt
- 1 egg
- ½ tablespoon paprika
- 1 teaspoon sesame oil

DIRECTIONS:

1. Put the ground turkey and ground chicken in a large bowl.
2. Sprinkle the meat with dried dill, ground coriander, almond flour, minced garlic, salt, and paprika.
3. Then chop the fresh spinach and add it to the ground poultry mixture.
4. break the egg into the meat mixture and mix well until you get a smooth texture.
5. Great the air fryer basket tray with the olive oil.
6. Preheat the air fryer to 350 F.
7. Roll the ground meat mixture gently to make the flat layer.
8. Put the butter in the center of the meat layer.
9. Make the shape of the meatloaf from the ground meat mixture. Use your fingertips for this step.
10. Place the meatloaf in the air fryer basket tray.
11. Cook for 25 minutes.
12. When the meatloaf is cooked allow it to rest before serving.

NUTRITION: Calories: 142 Fat: 9.8 g Carbs: 1.7g Protein: 13g

72. Turkey Meatballs with Dried Dill

Preparation Time: 15 minutes
Cooking Time: 11 minutes
Servings: 9
INGREDIENTS:

- 1-pound ground turkey
- 1 teaspoon chili flakes
- ¼ cup chicken stock
- 2 tablespoon dried dill
- 1 egg
- 1 teaspoon salt
- 1 teaspoon paprika
- 1 tablespoon coconut flour
- 2 tablespoons heavy cream
- 1 teaspoon olive oil

DIRECTIONS:

1. in a bowl, whisk the egg with a fork.
2. Add the ground turkey and chili flakes.
3. Sprinkle the mixture with dried dill, salt, paprika, coconut flour, and mix it up.
4. Make the meatballs from the ground turkey mixture.
5. Preheat the air fryer to 360 F.
6. Grease the air fryer basket tray with the olive oil.
7. Then put the meatballs inside.
8. Cook the meatballs for 6 minutes - for 3 minutes on each side.
9. Sprinkle the meatballs with the heavy cream.
10. Cook the meatballs for 5 minutes more.
11. When the turkey meatballs are cooked - let them rest for 2-3 minutes.

NUTRITION: Calories: 124 Fat: 7.9g Carbs: 1.2g Protein: 14.8g

73. Chicken Coconut Poppers

Preparation Time: 10 minutes
Cooking Time: 10 minutes
Servings: 6
INGREDIENTS:

- ½ cup coconut flour
- 1 teaspoon chili flakes
- 1 teaspoon ground black pepper
- 1 teaspoon garlic powder
- 11 oz. chicken breast, boneless, skinless
- 1 tablespoon olive oil

DIRECTIONS:

1. Cut the chicken breast into sizeable cubes and put them in a large bowl.
2. Sprinkle the chicken cubes with the chili flakes, ground black pepper, garlic powder, and stir them well using your hands.
3. After this, sprinkle the chicken cubes with the almond flour.
4. Shake the bowl with the chicken cubes gently to coat the meat.
5. Preheat the air fryer to 365 F.
6. Grease the air fryer basket tray with the olive oil.
7. Place the chicken cubes inside.
8. Cook the chicken poppers for 10 minutes.
9. Turn the chicken poppers over after 5 minutes of cooking.
10. Allow the cooked chicken poppers to cool before serving.

NUTRITION: Calories: 123 Fat: 4.6g Carbs: 6.9g Protein: 13.2g

74. Parmesan Beef Slices

Preparation Time: 14 minutes
Cooking Time: 25 minutes
Servings: 4
INGREDIENTS:

- 12 oz. beef brisket
- 1 teaspoon kosher salt
- 7 oz. Parmesan, sliced
- 5 oz. chive stems
- 1 teaspoon turmeric
- 1 teaspoon dried oregano
- 2 teaspoon butter

DIRECTIONS:

1. Slice the beef brisket into 4 slices.
2. Sprinkle every beef slice with the turmeric and dried oregano.
3. Grease the air fryer basket tray with the butter.
4. Put the beef slices inside.
5. Dice the chives.
6. Make a layer using the diced chives over the beef slices.
7. Then make a layer using the Parmesan cheese.
8. Preheat the air fryer to 365 F.
9. Cook the beef slices for 25 minutes.

NUTRITION: Calories: 348 Fat: 18g Carbs: 5g Protein: 42.1g

75. Chili Beef Jerky

Preparation Time: 25 minutes
Cooking Time: 2.5 hours
Servings: 6
INGREDIENTS:

- 14 oz. beef flank steak
- 1 teaspoon chili pepper
- 3 tablespoon apple cider vinegar
- 1 teaspoon ground black pepper
- 1 teaspoon onion powder
- 1 teaspoon garlic powder
- ¼ teaspoon liquid smoke

DIRECTIONS:

1. Slice the beefsteak into the medium strips and then tenderize each piece.
2. Take a bowl and combine the apple cider vinegar, ground black pepper, onion powder, garlic powder, and liquid smoke.
3. Whisk gently with a fork.
4. Then transfer the beef pieces in the mixture and stir well.
5. Leave the meat to marinade for up to 8 hours.
6. Put the marinated beef pieces in the air fryer rack.
7. Cook the beef jerky for 2.5 hours at 150 F.

NUTRITION: Calories: 129 Fat: 4.1g Carbs: 1.1g Protein: 20.2 g

76. Spinach Beef Heart

Preparation Time: 15 minutes
Cooking Time: 20 minutes
Servings: 4
INGREDIENTS:

- 1-pound beef heart
- 5 oz. chive stems
- ½ cup fresh spinach
- 1 teaspoon salt
- 1 teaspoon ground black pepper
- 3 cups chicken stock
- 1 teaspoon butter

DIRECTIONS:

1. Remove all the fat from the beef heart.
2. Dice the chives.
3. Chop the fresh spinach.
4. Combine the diced chives, fresh spinach, and butter together. Stir it.
5. Make a cut in the beef heart and fill it with the spinach-chives mixture.
6. Preheat the air fryer to 400 F.
7. Pour the chicken stock into the air fryer basket tray.
8. Sprinkle the Prepared stuffed beef heart with the salt and ground black pepper.
9. Put the beef heart in the air fryer and cook it for 20 minutes.
10. Remove the cooked heart from the air fryer and slice it.
11. Sprinkle the slices with the remaining liquid from the air fryer.

NUTRITION: Calories: 216 Fat: 6.8g Fiber: 0.8g Carbs: 3.8g Protein: 33.3

SIDE DISHES

77. Parmesan Sweet Potato Casserole

Preparation Time: 15 minutes
Cooking Time: 35 minutes
Servings: 2
INGREDIENTS:

- 2 sweet potatoes, peeled
- ½ yellow onion, sliced
- ½ cup cream
- ¼ cup spinach
- 2 oz. Parmesan cheese, shredded
- ½ teaspoon salt
- 1 tomato
- 1 teaspoon olive oil

DIRECTIONS:

1. Chop the sweet potatoes.
2. Chop the tomato.
3. Chop the spinach.
4. Spray the air fryer tray with the olive oil.
5. Then place on the layer of the chopped sweet potato.
6. Add the layer of the sliced onion.
7. After this, sprinkle the sliced onion with the chopped spinach and tomatoes.
8. Sprinkle the casserole with the salt and shredded cheese.
9. Pour cream.
10. Preheat the air fryer to 390 F.
11. Cover the air fryer tray with the foil.
12. Cook the casserole for 35 minutes.
13. When the casserole is cooked - serve it.
14. Enjoy!

NUTRITION: Calories: 93 Fat: 1.8g Fiber: 3.4g Carbs: 20.3g Protein: 1.8g

78. Spicy Zucchini Slices

Preparation Time: 10 minutes
Cooking Time: 6 minutes
Servings: 2
INGREDIENTS:

- 1 teaspoon cornstarch
- 1 zucchini
- ½ teaspoon chili flakes
- 1 tablespoon flour
- 1 egg
- ¼ teaspoon salt

DIRECTIONS:

1. Slice the zucchini and sprinkle with the chili flakes and salt.
2. Crack the egg into the bowl and whisk it.
3. Dip the zucchini slices in the whisked egg.
4. Combine together cornstarch with the flour. Stir it.
5. Coat the zucchini slices with the cornstarch mixture.
6. Preheat the air fryer to 400 F.
7. Place the zucchini slices in the air fryer tray.
8. Cook the zucchini slices for 4 minutes.
9. After this, flip the slices to another side and cook for 2 minutes more.
10. Serve the zucchini slices hot.
11. Enjoy!

NUTRITION: Calories: 67 Fat: 2.4g Fiber: 1.2g Carbs: 7.7g Protein: 4.4g

79. Cheddar Potato Gratin

Preparation Time: 15 minutes
Cooking Time: 20 minutes
Servings: 2
INGREDIENTS:

- 2 potatoes
- 1/3 cup half and half
- 1 tablespoon oatmeal flour
- ¼ teaspoon ground black pepper
- 1 egg
- 2 oz. Cheddar cheese

DIRECTIONS:

1. Wash the potatoes and slice them into thin pieces.
2. Preheat the air fryer to 365 F.
3. Put the potato slices in the air fryer and cook them for 10 minutes.
4. Meanwhile, combine the half and half, oatmeal flour, and ground black pepper.
5. Crack the egg into the liquid and whisk it carefully.
6. Shred Cheddar cheese.
7. When the potato is cooked – take 2 ramekins and place the potatoes on them.
8. Pour the half and half mixture.
9. Sprinkle the gratin with shredded Cheddar cheese.
10. Cook the gratin for 10 minutes at 360 F.
11. Serve the meal immediately.
12. Enjoy!

NUTRITION: Calories: 353 Fat: 16.6g Fiber: 5.4g Carbs: 37.2g Protein: 15g

80. Salty Lemon Artichokes

Preparation Time: 15 minutes
Cooking Time: 45 minutes
Servings: 2
INGREDIENTS:

- 1 lemon
- 2 artichokes
- 1 teaspoon kosher salt
- 1 garlic head
- 2 teaspoons olive oil

DIRECTIONS:

1. Cut off the edges of the artichokes.
2. Cut the lemon into the halves.
3. Peel the garlic head and chop the garlic cloves roughly.
4. Then place the chopped garlic in the artichokes.
5. Sprinkle the artichokes with the olive oil and kosher salt.
6. Then squeeze the lemon juice into the artichokes.
7. Wrap the artichokes in the foil.
8. Preheat the air fryer to 330 F.
9. Place the wrapped artichokes in the air fryer and cook for 45 minutes.
10. When the artichokes are cooked – discard the foil and serve.
11. Enjoy!

NUTRITION: Calories: 133 Fat: 5g Fiber: 9.7g Carbs: 21.7g Protein: 6g

81. Asparagus & Parmesan

Preparation Time: 10 minutes
Cooking Time: 6 minutes
Servings: 2
INGREDIENTS:

- 1 teaspoon sesame oil
- 11 oz. asparagus
- 1 teaspoon chicken stock
- ½ teaspoon ground white pepper
- 3 oz. Parmesan

DIRECTIONS:

1. Wash the asparagus and chop it roughly.
2. Sprinkle the chopped asparagus with the chicken stock and ground white pepper.
3. Then sprinkle the vegetables with the sesame oil and shake them.
4. Place the asparagus in the air fryer basket.
5. Cook the vegetables for 4 minutes at 400 F.
6. Meanwhile, shred Parmesan cheese.
7. When the time is over – shake the asparagus gently and sprinkle with the shredded cheese.
8. Cook the asparagus for 2 minutes more at 400 F.
9. After this, transfer the cooked asparagus in the serving plates.
10. Serve and taste it!

NUTRITION: Calories: 189 Fat: 11.6g Fiber: 3.4g Carbs: 7.9g Protein: 17.2g

82. Carrot Lentil Burgers

Preparation Time: 10 minutes
Cooking Time: 12 minutes
Servings: 2
INGREDIENTS:

- 6 oz. lentils, cooked
- 1 egg
- 2 oz. carrot, grated
- 1 teaspoon semolina
- ½ teaspoon salt
- 1 teaspoon turmeric
- 1 tablespoon butter

DIRECTIONS:

1. Crack the egg into the bowl and whisk it.
2. Add the cooked lentils and mash the mixture with the help of the fork.
3. Then sprinkle the mixture with the grated carrot, semolina, salt, and turmeric.
4. Mix it up and make the medium burgers.
5. Put the butter into the lentil burgers. It will make them juicy.
6. Preheat the air fryer to 360 F.
7. Put the lentil burgers in the air fryer and cook for 12 minutes.
8. Flip the burgers into another side after 6 minutes of cooking.
9. Then chill the cooked lentil burgers and serve them.
10. Enjoy!

NUTRITION: Calories: 404 Fat: 9g Fiber: 26.9g Carbs: 56g Protein: 25.3g

83. Corn on Cobs

Preparation Time: 10 minutes
Cooking Time: 10 minutes
Servings: 2
INGREDIENTS:

- 2 fresh corn on cobs
- 2 teaspoon butter
- 1 teaspoon salt
- 1 teaspoon paprika
- ¼ teaspoon olive oil

DIRECTIONS:

1. Preheat the air fryer to 400 F.
2. Rub the corn on cobs with the salt and paprika.
3. Then sprinkle the corn on cobs with the olive oil.
4. Place the corn on cobs in the air fryer basket.
5. Cook the corn on cobs for 10 minutes.
6. When the time is over – transfer the corn on cobs in the serving plates and rub with the butter gently.
7. Serve the meal immediately.
8. Enjoy!

NUTRITION: Calories: 122 Fat: 5.5g Fiber: 2.4g Carbs: 17.6g Protein: 3.2g

84. Sugary Carrot Strips

Preparation Time: 10 minutes
Cooking Time: 10 minutes
Servings: 2
INGREDIENTS:

- 2 carrots
- 1 teaspoon brown sugar
- 1 teaspoon olive oil
- 1 tablespoon soy sauce
- 1 teaspoon honey
- ½ teaspoon ground black pepper

DIRECTIONS:

1. Peel the carrot and cut it into the strips.
2. Then put the carrot strips in the bowl.
3. Sprinkle the carrot strips with the olive oil, soy sauce, honey, and ground black pepper.
4. Shake the mixture gently.
5. Preheat the air fryer to 360 F.
6. Cook the carrot for 10 minutes.
7. After this, shake the carrot strips well.
8. Enjoy!

NUTRITION: Calories: 67 Fat: 2.4g Fiber: 1.7g Carbs: 11.3g Protein: 1.1g

85. Onion Green Beans

Preparation Time: 10 minutes
Cooking Time: 12 minutes
Servings: 2
INGREDIENTS:

- 11 oz. green beans
- 1 tablespoon onion powder
- 1 tablespoon olive oil
- ½ teaspoon salt
- ¼ teaspoon chili flakes

DIRECTIONS:

1. Wash the green beans carefully and place them in the bowl.
2. Sprinkle the green beans with the onion powder, salt, chili flakes, and olive oil.
3. Shake the green beans carefully.
4. Preheat the air fryer to 400 F.
5. Put the green beans in the air fryer and cook for 8 minutes.
6. After this, shake the green beans and cook them for 4 minutes more at 400 F.
7. When the time is over – shake the green beans.
8. Serve the side dish and enjoy!

NUTRITION: Calories: 1205 Fat: 7.2g Fiber: 5.5g Carbs: 13.9g Protein: 3.2g

86. Mozzarella Radish Salad

Preparation Time: 10 minutes
Cooking Time: 20 minutes
Servings: 2
INGREDIENTS:

- 8 oz. radish
- 4 oz. Mozzarella
- 1 teaspoon balsamic vinegar
- ½ teaspoon salt
- 1 tablespoon olive oil
- 1 teaspoon dried oregano

DIRECTIONS:

1. Wash the radish carefully and cut it into the halves.
2. Preheat the air fryer to 360 F.
3. Put the radish halves in the air fryer basket.
4. Sprinkle the radish with the salt and olive oil.
5. Cook the radish for 20 minutes.
6. Shake the radish after 10 minutes of cooking.
7. When the time is over – transfer the radish to the serving plate.
8. Chop Mozzarella roughly.
9. Sprinkle the radish with Mozzarella, balsamic vinegar, and dried oregano.
10. Stir it gently with the help of 2 forks.
11. Serve it immediately.

NUTRITION: Calories: 241 Fat: 17.2g Fiber: 2.1g Carbs: 6.4g Protein: 16.9g

87. Cremini Mushroom Satay

Preparation Time: 10 minutes
Cooking Time: 6 minutes
Servings: 2
INGREDIENTS:

- 7 oz. cremini mushrooms
- 2 tablespoon coconut milk
- 1 tablespoon butter
- 1 teaspoon chili flakes
- ½ teaspoon balsamic vinegar
- ½ teaspoon curry powder
- ½ teaspoon white pepper

DIRECTIONS:

1. Wash the mushrooms carefully.
2. Then sprinkle the mushrooms with the chili flakes, curry powder, and white pepper.
3. Preheat the air fryer to 400 F.
4. Toss the butter in the air fryer basket and melt it.
5. Put the mushrooms in the air fryer and cook for 2 minutes.
6. Shake the mushrooms well and sprinkle with the coconut milk and balsamic vinegar.
7. Cook the mushrooms for 4 minutes more at 400 F.
8. Then skewer the mushrooms on the wooden sticks and serve.
9. Enjoy!

NUTRITION: Calories 116 Fat: 9.5g Fiber: 1.3g Carbs: 5.6g Protein: 3g

88. Eggplant Ratatouille

Preparation Time: 15 minutes
Cooking Time: 15 minutes
Servings: 2
INGREDIENTS:

- 1 eggplant
- 1 sweet yellow pepper
- 3 cherry tomatoes
- 1/3 white onion, chopped
- ½ teaspoon garlic clove, sliced
- 1 teaspoon olive oil
- ½ teaspoon ground black pepper
- ½ teaspoon Italian seasoning

DIRECTIONS:

1. Preheat the air fryer to 360 F.
2. Peel the eggplants and chop them.
3. Put the chopped eggplants in the air fryer basket.
4. Chop the cherry tomatoes and add them to the air fryer basket.
5. Then add chopped onion, sliced garlic clove, olive oil, ground black pepper, and Italian seasoning.
6. Chop the sweet yellow pepper roughly and add it to the air fryer basket.
7. Shake the vegetables gently and cook for 15 minutes.
8. Stir the meal after 8 minutes of cooking.
9. Transfer the cooked ratatouille in the serving plates.
10. Enjoy!

NUTRITION: Calories: 149 Fat: 3.7g Fiber: 11.7g Carbs: 28.9g Protein: 5.1g

89. Cheddar Portobello Mushrooms

Preparation Time: 15 minutes
Cooking Time: 6 minutes
Servings: 2
INGREDIENTS:

- 2 Portobello mushroom hats
- 2 slices Cheddar cheese
- ¼ cup panko breadcrumbs
- ½ teaspoon salt
- ½ teaspoon ground black pepper
- 1 egg
- 1 teaspoon oatmeal
- 2 oz. bacon, chopped cooked

DIRECTIONS:

1. Crack the egg into the bowl and whisk it.
2. Combine the ground black pepper, oatmeal, salt, and breadcrumbs in the separate bowl.
3. Dip the mushroom hats in the whisked egg.
4. After this, coat the mushroom hats in the breadcrumb mixture.
5. Preheat the air fryer to 400 F.
6. Place the mushrooms in the air fryer basket tray and cook for 3 minutes.
7. After this, put the chopped bacon and sliced cheese over the mushroom hats and cook the meal for 3 minutes.
8. When the meal is cooked – let it chill gently.
9. Enjoy!

NUTRITION: Calories: 376 Fat: 24.1g Fiber: 1.8g Carbs: 14.6g Protein: 25.2g

SEAFOODS

90. Coconut Salsa on Chipotle Fish Tacos

Preparation Time: 10 minutes
Cooking Time: 10 minutes
Servings: 4
INGREDIENTS:

- ¼ cup chopped fresh cilantro
- ½ cup seeded and finely chopped plum tomato
- 1 cup peeled and finely chopped mango
- 1 lime cut into wedges
- 1 tablespoon chipotle Chile powder
- 1 tablespoon safflower oil
- 1/3 cup finely chopped red onion
- 10 tablespoon fresh lime juice, divided
- 4 6-oz boneless, skinless cod fillets
- 5 tablespoon dried unsweetened shredded coconut
- 8 pcs of 6-inch tortillas, heated

DIRECTIONS:

1. Whisk well Chile powder, oil, and 4 tablespoon lime juice in a glass baking dish. Add cod and marinate for 12 – 15 minutes. Turning once halfway through the marinating time.
2. Make the salsa by mixing coconut, 6 tablespoon lime juice, cilantro, onions, tomatoes and mangoes in a medium bowl. Set aside.
3. On high, heat a grill pan. Place cod and grill for four minutes per side turning only once.
4. Once cooked, slice cod into large flakes and evenly divide onto tortilla.
5. Evenly divide salsa on top of cod and serve with a side of lime wedges.

NUTRITION: Calories: 477 Protein: 35.0g Fat: 12.4g Carbs: 57.4g

91. Baked Cod Crusted with Herbs

Preparation Time: 5 minutes
Cooking Time: 10 minutes
Servings: 4
INGREDIENTS:

- ¼ cup honey
- ¼ teaspoon salt
- ½ cup panko
- ½ teaspoon pepper
- 1 tablespoon extra virgin olive oil
- 1 tablespoon lemon juice
- 1 teaspoon dried basil
- 1 teaspoon dried parsley
- 1 teaspoon rosemary
- 4 pieces of 4-oz cod fillets

DIRECTIONS:

1. With olive oil, grease a 9 x 13-inch baking pan and preheat oven to 375oF.
2. In a zip top bag mix panko, rosemary, salt, pepper, parsley and basil.
3. Evenly spread cod fillets in prepped dish and drizzle with lemon juice.
4. Then brush the fillets with honey on all sides. Discard remaining honey if any.
5. Then evenly divide the panko mixture on top of cod fillets.
6. Pop in the oven and bake for ten minutes or until fish is cooked.
7. Serve and enjoy.

NUTRITION: Calories: 137 Protein: 5g Fat: 2g Carbs: 21g

92. Cajun Garlic Shrimp Noodle Bowl

Preparation Time: 10 minutes
Cooking Time: 15 minutes
Servings: 2
INGREDIENTS:

- ½ teaspoon salt
- 1 onion, sliced
- 1 red pepper, sliced
- 1 tablespoon butter
- 1 teaspoon garlic granules
- 1 teaspoon onion powder
- 1 teaspoon paprika
- 2 large zucchinis, cut into noodle strips
- 20 jumbo shrimps, shells removed and deveined
- 3 cloves garlic, minced
- 3 tablespoon ghee
- A dash of cayenne pepper
- A dash of red pepper flakes

DIRECTIONS:

1. Prepare the Cajun seasoning by mixing the onion powder, garlic granules, pepper flakes, cayenne pepper, paprika and salt. Toss in the shrimp to coat in the seasoning.
2. In a skillet, heat the ghee and sauté the garlic. Add in the red pepper and onions and continue sautéing for 4 minutes.
3. Add the Cajun shrimp and cook until opaque. Set aside.
4. In another pan, heat the butter and sauté the zucchini noodles for three minutes.
5. Assemble by the placing the Cajun shrimps on top of the zucchini noodles.

NUTRITION: Calories: 712 Fat: 30.0g Protein: 97.8g Carbs: 20.2g

93. Crazy Saganaki Shrimp

Preparation Time: 10 minutes
Cooking Time: 10 minutes
Servings: 4
INGREDIENTS:

- ¼ teaspoon salt
- ½ cup Chardonnay
- ½ cup crumbled Greek feta cheese
- 1 medium bulb. fennel, cored and finely chopped
- 1 small Chile pepper, seeded and minced
- 1 tablespoon extra virgin olive oil
- 12 jumbo shrimps, deveined with tails left on
- 2 tablespoon lemon juice, divided
- 5 scallions sliced thinly
- Pepper to taste

DIRECTIONS:

1. In medium bowl, mix salt, lemon juice and shrimp.
2. On medium fire, place a saganaki pan (or large nonstick saucepan) and heat oil.
3. Sauté Chile pepper, scallions, and fennel for 4 minutes or until starting to brown and is already soft.
4. Add wine and sauté for another minute.
5. Place shrimps on top of fennel, cover and cook for 4 minutes or until shrimps are pink.
6. Remove just the shrimp and transfer to a plate.
7. Add pepper, feta and 1 tablespoon lemon juice to pan and cook for a minute or until cheese begins to melt.
8. To serve, place cheese and fennel mixture on a serving plate and top with shrimps.

NUTRITION: Calories: 310 Protein: 49.7g Fat: 6.8g Carbs: 8.4g

94. Creamy Bacon-Fish Chowder

Preparation Time: 10 minutes
Cooking Time: 30 minutes
Servings: 8
INGREDIENTS:

- 1 1/2 lbs. cod
- 1 1/2 teaspoon dried thyme
- 1 large onion, chopped
- 1 medium carrot, coarsely chopped
- 1 tablespoon butter, cut into small pieces
- 1 teaspoon salt, divided
- 3 1/2 cups baking potato, peeled and cubed
- 3 slices uncooked bacon
- 3/4 teaspoon ground black pepper, divided
- 4 1/2 cups water
- 4 bay leaves
- 4 cups 2% reduced-fat milk

DIRECTIONS:

1. In a large skillet, add the water and bay leaves and let it simmer. Add the fish. Cover and let it simmer some more until the flesh flakes easily with fork. Remove the fish from the skillet and cut into large pieces. Set aside the cooking liquid.
2. Place Dutch oven in medium heat and cook the bacon until crisp. Remove the bacon and reserve the bacon drippings. Crush the bacon and set aside.
3. Stir potato, onion and carrot in the pan with the bacon drippings, cook over medium heat for 10 minutes. Add the cooking liquid, bay leaves, 1/2 teaspoon salt, 1/4 teaspoon pepper and thyme, let it boil. Lower the heat and let simmer for 11 minutes. Add the milk and butter, simmer until the potatoes becomes tender, but do not boil. Add the fish, 1/2 teaspoon salt, 1/2 teaspoon pepper. Remove the bay leaves.
4. Serve sprinkled with the crushed bacon.

NUTRITION: Calories: 400 Carbs: 34.5g Protein: 20.8g Fat: 19.7g

95. Crisped Coco-Shrimp with Mango Dip

Preparation Time: 10 minutes
Cooking Time: 20 minutes
Servings: 4
INGREDIENTS:

- 1 cup shredded coconut
- 1 lb. raw shrimp, peeled and deveined
- 2 egg whites
- 4 tablespoon tapioca starch
- Pepper and salt to taste
- Mango Dip Ingredients:
- 1 cup mango, chopped
- 1 jalapeño, thinly minced
- 1 teaspoon lime juice
- 1/3 cup coconut milk
- 3 teaspoon raw honey

DIRECTIONS:

1. Preheat oven to 400oF.
2. Ready a pan with wire rack on top.
3. In a medium bowl, add tapioca starch and season with pepper and salt.
4. In a second medium bowl, add egg whites and whisk.
5. In a third medium bowl, add coconut.
6. To ready shrimps, dip first in tapioca starch, then egg whites, and then coconut. Place dredged shrimp on wire rack. Repeat until all shrimps are covered.
7. Pop shrimps in the oven and roast for 10 minutes per side.
8. Meanwhile make the dip by adding all ingredients in a blender. Puree until smooth and creamy. Transfer to a dipping bowl.
9. Once shrimps are golden brown, serve with mango dip.

NUTRITION: Calories: 294.2 Protein: 26.6g Fat: 7g Carbs: 31.2g

96. Cucumber-Basil Salsa on Halibut Pouches

Preparation Time: 10 minutes
Cooking Time: 17 minutes
Servings: 4
INGREDIENTS:

- 1 lime, thinly sliced into 8 pieces
- 2 cups mustard greens, stems removed
- 2 teaspoon olive oil
- 4 – 5 radishes trimmed and quartered
- 4 4-oz skinless halibut filets
- 4 large fresh basil leaves
- Cayenne pepper to taste – optional
- Pepper and salt to taste
- Salsa Ingredients:
- 1 ½ cups diced cucumber
- 1 ½ finely chopped fresh basil leaves
- 2 teaspoon fresh lime juice
- Pepper and salt to taste

DIRECTIONS:

1. Preheat oven to 400°F.
2. Prepare parchment papers by making 4 pieces of 15 x 12-inch rectangles. Lengthwise, fold in half and unfold pieces on the table.
3. Season halibut fillets with pepper, salt and cayenne—if using cayenne.
4. Just to the right of the fold, place ½ cup of mustard greens. Add a basil leaf on center of mustard greens and topped with 1 lime slice. Around the greens, layer ¼ of the radishes. Drizzle with ½ teaspoon of oil, season with pepper and salt. Top it with a slice of halibut fillet.
5. Just as you would make a calzone, fold parchment paper over your filling and crimp the edges of the parchment paper beginning from one end to the other end. To seal the end of the crimped parchment paper, pinch it.
6. Repeat process to remaining ingredients until you have 4 pieces of parchment papers filled with halibut and greens.
7. Place pouches in a pan and bake in the oven until halibut is flaky, around 15 to 17 minutes.
8. While waiting for halibut pouches to cook, make your salsa by mixing all salsa ingredients in a medium bowl.
9. Once halibut is cooked, remove from oven and make a tear on top. Be careful of the steam as it is very hot. Equally divide salsa and spoon ¼ of salsa on top of halibut through the slit you have created.

NUTRITION: Calories: 335.4 Protein: 20.2g Fat: 16.3g Carbs: 22.1g

97. Curry Salmon with Mustard

Preparation Time: 10 minutes
Cooking Time: 8 minutes
Servings: 4
INGREDIENTS:

- ¼ teaspoon ground red pepper or chili powder
- ¼ teaspoon ground turmeric
- ¼ teaspoon salt
- 1 teaspoon honey
- 1/8 teaspoon garlic powder or a minced clove garlic
- 2 teaspoon. whole grain mustard
- 4 pcs 6-oz salmon fillets

Directions:

1. In a small bowl mix well salt, garlic powder, red pepper, turmeric, honey and mustard.
2. Preheat oven to broil and grease a baking dish with cooking spray.
3. Place salmon on baking dish with skin side down and spread evenly mustard mixture on top of salmon.
4. Pop in the oven and broil until flaky around 8 minutes.

NUTRITION: Calories: 324 Fat: 18.9 g Protein: 34 g Carbs: 2.9 g

98. Dijon Mustard and Lime Marinated Shrimp

Preparation Time: 10 minutes
Cooking Time: 10 minutes
Servings: 8
INGREDIENTS:

- ½ cup fresh lime juice, and lime zest as garnish
- ½ cup rice vinegar
- ½ teaspoon hot sauce
- 1 bay leaf
- 1 cup water
- 1 lb. uncooked shrimp, peeled and deveined
- 1 medium red onion, chopped
- 2 tablespoon capers
- 2 tablespoon Dijon mustard
- 3 whole cloves

DIRECTIONS:

1. Mix hot sauce, mustard, capers, lime juice and onion in a shallow baking dish and set aside.
2. Bring to a boil in a large saucepan bay leaf, cloves, vinegar and water.
3. Once boiling, add shrimps and cook for a minute while stirring continuously.
4. Drain shrimps and pour shrimps into onion mixture.
5. For an hour, refrigerate while covered the shrimps.
6. Then serve shrimps cold and garnished with lime zest.

NUTRITION: Calories: 232.2 Protein: 17.8g Fat: 3g Carbs: 15g

99. Dill Relish on White Sea Bass

Preparation Time: 10 minutes
Cooking Time: 12 minutes
Servings: 4
INGREDIENTS:

- 1 ½ tablespoon chopped white onion
- 1 ½ teaspoon chopped fresh dill
- 1 lemon, quartered
- 1 teaspoon Dijon mustard
- 1 teaspoon lemon juice
- 1 teaspoon pickled baby capers, drained
- 4 pieces of 4-oz white sea bass fillets

DIRECTIONS:

1. Preheat oven to 375°F.
2. Mix lemon juice, mustard, dill, capers and onions in a small bowl.
3. Prepare four aluminum foil squares and place 1 fillet per foil.
4. Squeeze a lemon wedge per fish.
5. Evenly divide into 4 the dill spread and drizzle over fillet.
6. Close the foil over the fish securely and pop in the oven.
7. Bake for 12 minutes or until fish is cooked through.
8. Remove from foil and transfer to a serving platter, serve and enjoy.

NUTRITION: Calories: 115 Protein: 7g Fat: 1g Carbs: 12g

LEAN AND GREEN RECIPES

100. Tomatillo and Green Chili Pork Stew

Preparation Time: 10 minutes
Cooking Time: 20 minutes
Servings: 4
INGREDIENTS:

- 2 scallions, chopped
- 2 cloves of garlic
- 1 lb. tomatillos, trimmed and chopped
- 8 large romaine or green lettuce leaves, divided
- 2 serrano chilies, seeds, and membranes
- ½ tsp of dried Mexican oregano (or you can use regular oregano)
- 1 ½ lb. of boneless pork loin, to be cut into bite-sized cubes
- ¼ cup of cilantro, chopped
- ¼ tablespoon (each) salt and paper
- 1 jalapeno, seeds and membranes to be removed and thinly sliced
- 1 cup of sliced radishes
- 4 lime wedges

DIRECTIONS:

1. Combine scallions, garlic, tomatillos, 4 lettuce leaves, serrano chilies, and oregano in a blender. Then puree until smooth
2. Put pork and tomatillo mixture in a medium pot. 1-inch of puree should cover the pork; if not, add water until it covers it. Season with pepper & salt, and cover it simmers. Simmer on heat for approximately 20 minutes.
3. Now, finely shred the remaining lettuce leaves.
4. When the stew is done cooking, garnish with cilantro, radishes, finely shredded lettuce, sliced jalapenos, and lime wedges.

NUTRITION: Calories: 370 Protein: 36g Carbohydrate: 14g Fat: 19 g

101. Optavia Cloud Bread

Preparation Time: 25 minutes
Cooking Time: 35 minutes
Servings: 3
INGREDIENTS:

- ½ cup of Fat-free 0% Plain Greek Yogurt (4.4 0z)
- 3 Eggs, Separated
- 16 teaspoon Cream of Tartar
- 1 Packet sweetener (a granulated sweetener just like stevia)

DIRECTIONS:

1. For about 30 minutes before making this meal, place the Kitchen Aid Bowl and the whisk attachment in the freezer.
2. Preheat your oven to 30 degrees
3. Remove the mixing bowl and whisk attachment from the freezer
4. Separate the eggs. Now put the egg whites in the Kitchen Aid Bowl, and they should be in a different medium-sized bowl.
5. In the medium-sized bowl containing the yolks, mix in the sweetener and yogurt.
6. In the bowl containing the egg white, add in the cream of tartar. Beat this mixture until the egg whites turn to stiff peaks.
7. Now, take the egg yolk mixture and carefully fold it into the egg whites. Be cautious and avoid over-stirring.
8. Place baking paper on a baking tray and spray with cooking spray.
9. Scoop out 6 equally-sized "blobs" of the "dough" onto the parchment paper.
10. Bake for about 25-35 minutes (make sure you check when it is 25 minutes, in some ovens, they are done at this timestamp). You will know they are done as they will get brownish at the top and have some crack.
11. Most people like them cold against being warm
12. Most people like to re-heat in a toast oven or toaster to get them a little bit crispy.
13. Your serving size should be about 2 pieces.

NUTRITION: Calories: 234 Protein: 23g Carbs: 5g Fiber: 8g Sodium: 223g

102. Avocado Lime Shrimp Salad

Preparation Time: 15 minutes
Cooking Time: 0 minutes
Servings: 2
INGREDIENTS:

- 14 ounces of jumbo cooked shrimp, peeled and deveined; chopped
- 4 ½ ounces of avocado, diced
- 1 ½ cup of tomato, diced
- ¼ cup of chopped green onion
- ¼ cup of jalapeno with the seeds removed, diced fine
- 1 teaspoon of olive oil
- 2 tablespoons of lime juice
- 1/8 teaspoon of salt
- 1 tablespoon of chopped cilantro

DIRECTIONS:

1. Get a small bowl and combine green onion, olive oil, lime juice, pepper, a pinch of salt. Wait for about 5 minutes for all of them to marinate and mellow the flavor of the onion.
2. Get a large bowl and combined chopped shrimp, tomato, avocado, jalapeno. Combine all of the ingredients, add cilantro, and gently toss.
3. Add pepper and salt as desired.

NUTRITION: Calories: 314 Protein: 26g Carbs: 15g Fiber: 9g

103. Broccoli Cheddar Breakfast Bake

Preparation Time: 10 minutes
Cooking Time: 45 minutes
Servings: 4
INGREDIENTS:

- 9 eggs
- 6 cups of small broccoli florets
- ¼ teaspoon of salt
- 1 cup of unsweetened almond milk
- ¼ teaspoon of cayenne pepper
- ¼ teaspoon of ground pepper
- Cooking spray
- 4 oz. of shredded, reduced-fat cheddar

DIRECTIONS:

1. Preheat your oven to about 375 degrees
2. In your large microwave-safe, add broccoli and 2 to 3 tablespoon of water. Microwave on high heat for 4 minutes or until it becomes tender. Now transfer the broccoli to a colander to drain excess liquid
3. Get a medium-sized bowl and whisk the milk, eggs, and seasonings together.
4. Set the broccoli neatly on the bottom of a lightly greased 13 x 9-inch baking dish. Sprinkle the cheese gently on the broccoli and pour the egg mixture on top of it.
5. Bake for about 45 minutes or until the center is set and the top forms a light brown crust.

NUTRITION: Calories: 290 Protein: 25g Carbohydrate: 8g Fat: 18 g

104. Grilled Mahi Mahi with Jicama Slaw

Preparation Time: 20 minutes
Cooking Time: 10 minutes
Servings: 4
INGREDIENTS:

- 1 teaspoon each for pepper and salt, divided
- 1 tablespoon of lime juice, divided
- 2 tablespoon + 2 teaspoons of extra virgin olive oil
- 4 raw mahi-mahi fillets, which should be about 8 oz. each
- ½ cucumber which should be thinly cut into long strips like matchsticks (it should yield about 1 cup)
- 1 jicama, which should be thinly cut into long strips like matchsticks (it should yield about 3 cups)
- 1 cup of alfalfa sprouts
- 2 cups of coarsely chopped watercress

DIRECTIONS:

1. Combine ½ teaspoon of both pepper and salt, 1 teaspoon of lime juice, and 2 teaspoons of oil in a small bowl. Then brush the mahi-mahi fillets all through with the olive oil mixture.
2. Grill the mahi-mahi on medium-high heat until it becomes done in about 5 minutes, turn it to the other side, and let it be done for about 5 minutes. (You will have an internal temperature of about 145°F).
3. For the slaw, combine the watercress, cucumber, jicama, and alfalfa sprouts in a bowl. Now combine ½ teaspoon of both pepper and salt, 2 teaspoons of lime juice, and 2 tablespoons of extra virgin oil in a small bowl. Drizzle it over slaw and toss together to combine.

NUTRITION: Calories: 320 Protein: 44g Carbohydrate: 10g Fat: 11 g

105. Rosemary Cauliflower Rolls

Preparation Time: 10 minutes
Cooking Time: 30 minutes
Servings: 3
INGREDIENTS:

- 1/3 cup of almond flour
- 4 cups of riced cauliflower
- 1/3 cup of reduced-fat, shredded mozzarella or cheddar cheese
- 2 eggs
- 2 tablespoon of fresh rosemary, finely chopped
- ½ teaspoon of salt

DIRECTIONS:

1. Preheat your oven to 400°F
2. Combine all the listed ingredients in a medium-sized bowl
3. Scoop cauliflower mixture into 12 evenly-sized rolls/biscuits onto a lightly-greased and foil-lined baking sheet.
4. Bake until it turns golden brown, which should be achieved in about 30 minutes.

Note: if you want to have the outside of the rolls/biscuits crisp, then broil for some minutes before serving.
NUTRITION: Calories: 254 Protein: 24g Carbohydrate: 7g Fat: 8 g

106. Mediterranean Chicken Salad

Preparation Time: 5 minutes
Cooking Time: 25 minutes
Servings: 4
INGREDIENTS:

- For Chicken:
- 1 ¾ lb. boneless, skinless chicken breast
- ¼ teaspoon each of pepper and salt (or as desired)
- 1 ½ tablespoon of butter, melted
- For Mediterranean salad:
- 1 cup of sliced cucumber
- 6 cups of romaine lettuce, that is torn or roughly chopped
- 10 pitted Kalamata olives
- 1 pint of cherry tomatoes
- 1/3 cup of reduced-fat feta cheese
- ¼ teaspoon each of pepper and salt (or lesser)
- 1 small lemon juice (it should be about 2 tablespoons)

DIRECTIONS:

1. Preheat your oven or grill to about 350°F.
2. Season the chicken with salt, butter, and black pepper
3. Roast or grill chicken until it reaches an internal temperature of 165°F in about 25 minutes. Once your chicken breasts are cooked, remove and keep aside to rest for about 5 minutes before you slice it.
4. Combine all the salad ingredients you have and toss everything together very well
5. Serve the chicken with Mediterranean salad

NUTRITION: Calories: 340 Protein: 45g Carbohydrate: 9g Fat: 4 g

107. Instant Pot Chipotle Chicken & Cauliflower Rice Bowls

Preparation Time: 10 minutes
Cooking Time: 20 minutes
Servings: 4
INGREDIENTS:

- 1/3 cup of salsa
- 1 quantity of 14.5 oz. of can fire-roasted diced tomatoes
- 1 canned chipotle pepper + 1 teaspoon sauce
- ½ teaspoon of dried oregano
- 1 teaspoon of cumin
- 1 ½ lb. of boneless, skinless chicken breast
- ¼ teaspoon of salt
- 1 cup of reduced-fat shredded Mexican cheese blend
- 4 cups of frozen riced cauliflower
- ½ medium-sized avocado, sliced

DIRECTIONS:

1. Combine the first ingredients in a blender and blend until they become smooth
2. Place chicken inside your instant pot, and pour the sauce over it. Cover the lid and close the pressure valve. Set it to 20 minutes at high temperature. Let the pressure release on its own before opening. Remove the piece and the chicken and then add it back to the sauce.
3. Microwave the riced cauliflower according to the directions on the package
4. Before you serve, divide the riced cauliflower, cheese, avocado, and chicken equally among the 4 bowls.

NUTRITION: Calories: 287 Protein: 35g Carbohydrate: 19g Fat: 12 g

108. Lemon Garlic Oregano Chicken with Asparagus

Preparation Time: 5 minutes
Cooking Time: 40 minutes
Servings: 4
INGREDIENTS:

- 1 small lemon, juiced (this should be about 2 tablespoons of lemon juice)
- 1 ¾ lb. of bone-in, skinless chicken thighs
- 2 tablespoon of fresh oregano, minced
- 2 cloves of garlic, minced
- 2 lbs. of asparagus, trimmed
- ¼ teaspoon each or less for black pepper and salt

DIRECTIONS:

1. Preheat the oven to about 350°F.
2. Put the chicken in a medium-sized bowl. Now, add the garlic, oregano, lemon juice, pepper, and salt and toss together to combine.
3. Roast the chicken in the airfryer oven until it reaches an internal temperature of 165°F in about 40 minutes. Once the chicken thighs have been cooked, remove and keep aside to rest.
4. Now, steam the asparagus on a stovetop or in a microwave to the desired doneness.
5. Serve asparagus with the roasted chicken thighs.

NUTRITION: Calories: 350 Fat: 10 g Carbohydrate: 10 g Protein: 32 g

109. Sheet Pan Chicken Fajita Lettuce Wraps

Preparation Time: 15 minutes
Cooking Time: 30 minutes
Servings: 2
INGREDIENTS:

- 1 lb. chicken breast, thinly sliced into strips
- 2 teaspoon of olive oil
- 2 bell peppers, thinly sliced into strips
- 2 teaspoon of fajita seasoning
- 6 leaves from a romaine heart
- Juice of half a lime
- ¼ cup plain of non-fat Greek yogurt

DIRECTIONS:

1. Preheat your oven to about 400°F
2. Combine all of the ingredients except for lettuce in a large plastic bag that can be resealed. Mix very well to coat vegetables and chicken with oil and seasoning evenly.
3. Spread the contents of the bag evenly on a foil-lined baking sheet. Bake it for about25-30 minutes, until the chicken is thoroughly cooked.
4. Serve on lettuce leaves and topped with Greek yogurt if you like

NUTRITION: Calories: 387 Fat: 6 g Carbohydrate: 14 g Protein: 18 g

110. Savory Cilantro Salmon

Preparation Time: 10 minutes
Cooking Time: 30 minutes
Servings: 4
INGREDIENTS:

- 2 tablespoons of fresh lime or lemon
- 4 cups of fresh cilantro, divided
- 2 tablespoon of hot red pepper sauce
- ½ teaspoon of salt. Divided
- 1 teaspoon of cumin
- 4, 7 oz. of salmon filets
- ½ cup of (4 oz.) water
- 2 cups of sliced red bell pepper
- 2 cups of sliced yellow bell pepper
- 2 cups of sliced green bell pepper
- Cooking spray
- ½ teaspoon of pepper

DIRECTIONS:

1. Get a blender or food processor and combine half of the cilantro, lime juice or lemon, cumin, hot red pepper sauce, water, and salt; then puree until they become smooth. Transfer the marinade gotten into a large re-sealable plastic bag.
2. Add salmon to marinade. Seal the bag, squeeze out air that might have been trapped inside, turn to coat salmon. Refrigerate for about 1 hour, turning as often as possible.
3. Now, after marinating, preheat your oven to about 400°F. Arrange the pepper slices in a single layer in a slightly-greased, medium-sized square baking dish. Bake it for 20 minutes, turn the pepper slices once.
4. Drain your salmon and do away with the marinade. Crust the upper part of the salmon with the remaining chopped, fresh cilantro. Place salmon on the top of the pepper slices and bake for about 12-14 minutes until you observe that the fish flakes easily when it is being tested with a fork
5. Enjoy

NUTRITION: Calories: 350 Carbohydrate: 15 g Protein: 42 g Fat: 13 g

111. Salmon Florentine

Preparation Time: 5 minutes
Cooking Time: 30 minutes
Servings: 4
INGREDIENTS:

- 1 ½ cups of chopped cherry tomatoes
- ½ cup of chopped green onions
- 2 garlic cloves, minced
- 1 teaspoon of olive oil
- 1 quantity of 12 oz. package frozen chopped spinach, thawed and patted dry
- ¼ teaspoon of crushed red pepper flakes
- ½ cup of part-skim ricotta cheese
- ¼ teaspoon each for pepper and salt
- 4 quantities of 5 ½ oz. wild salmon fillets
- Cooking spray

DIRECTIONS:

1. Preheat the oven to 350°F
2. Get a medium skillet to cook onions in oil until they start to soften, which should be in about 2 minutes. You can then add garlic inside the skillet and cook for an extra 1 minute. Add the spinach, red pepper flakes, tomatoes, pepper, and salt. Cook for 2 minutes while stirring. Remove the pan from the heat and let it cool for about 10 minutes. Stir in the ricotta
3. Put a quarter of the spinach mixture on top of each salmon fillet. Place the fillets on a slightly-greased rimmed baking sheet and bake it for 15 minutes or until you are sure that the salmon has been thoroughly cooked.

NUTRITION: Calories: 350 Carbohydrate: 15 g Protein: 42 g Fat: 13

112. Tomato Braised Cauliflower with Chicken

Preparation Time: 10 minutes
Cooking Time: 30 minutes
Servings: 4
INGREDIENTS:

- 4 garlic cloves, sliced
- 3 scallions, to be trimmed and cut into 1-inch pieces
- ¼ teaspoon of dried oregano
- ¼ teaspoon of crushed red pepper flakes
- 4 ½ cups of cauliflower
- 1 ½ cups of diced canned tomatoes
- 1 cup of fresh basil, gently torn
- ½ teaspoon each of pepper and salt, divided
- 1 ½ teaspoon of olive oil
- 1 ½ lb. of boneless, skinless chicken breasts

DIRECTIONS:

1. Get a saucepan and combine the garlic, scallions, oregano, crushed red pepper, cauliflower, and tomato, and add ¼ cup of water. Get everything boil together and add ¼ teaspoon of pepper and salt for seasoning, then cover the pot with a lid. Let it simmer for 10 minutes and stir as often as possible until you observe that the cauliflower is tender. Now, wrap up the seasoning with the remaining ¼ teaspoon of pepper and salt.
2. Toss the chicken breast with oil, olive prefebrably and let it roast in the oven with the heat of 450°F for 20 minutes and an internal temperature of 165°F. Allow the chicken to rest for like 10 minutes.
3. Now slice the chicken, and serve on a bed of tomato braised cauliflower.

NUTRITION: Calories: 290 Fat: 10 g Carbohydrate: 13 g Protein: 38 g

113. Cheeseburger Soup

Preparation Time: 20 minutes
Cooking Time: 25 minutes
Servings: 4
INGREDIENTS:

- ¼ cup of chopped onion
- 1 quantity of 14.5 oz. can diced tomato
- 1 lb. of 90% lean ground beef
- ¾ cup of diced celery
- 2 teaspoon of Worcestershire sauce
- 3 cups of low sodium chicken broth
- ¼ teaspoon of salt
- 1 teaspoon of dried parsley
- 7 cups of baby spinach
- ¼ teaspoon of ground pepper
- 4 oz. of reduced-fat shredded cheddar cheese

DIRECTIONS:

1. Get a large soup pot and cook the beef until it becomes brown. Add the celery, onion, and sauté until it becomes tender. Remove from the fire and drain excess liquid.
2. Stir in the broth, tomatoes, parsley, Worcestershire sauce, pepper, and salt. Cover and allow it to simmer on low heat for about 20 minutes
3. Add spinach and leave it to cook until it becomes wilted in about 1-3 minutes. Top each of your servings with 1 ounce of cheese.

NUTRITION: Calories: 400 Carbohydrate: 11 g Protein: 44 g Fat: 20 g

114. Braised Collard Greens in Peanut Sauce with Pork Tenderloin

Preparation Time: 20 minutes
Cooking Time: 1 hour 12 minutes
Servings: 4
INGREDIENTS:

- 2 cups of chicken stock
- 12 cups of chopped collard greens
- 5 tablespoon of powdered peanut butter
- 3 cloves of garlic, crushed
- 1 teaspoon of salt
- ½ teaspoon of allspice
- ½ teaspoon of black pepper
- 2 teaspoon of lemon juice
- ¾ teaspoon of hot sauce
- 1 ½ lb. of pork tenderloin

DIRECTIONS:

1. Get a pot with a tight-fitting lid and combine the collards with the garlic, chicken stock, hot sauce, and half of the pepper and salt. Cook on low heat for about 1 hour or until the collards become tender.
2. Once the collards are tender, stir in the allspice, lemon juice. And powdered peanut butter. Keep warm.
3. Season the pork tenderloin with the remaining pepper and salt, and broil in a toaster oven for 10 minutes when you have an internal temperature of 145°F. Make sure to turn the tenderloin every 2 minutes to achieve an even browning all over. After that, you can take away the pork from the oven and allow it to rest for like 5 minutes.
4. Slice the pork as you will

NUTRITION: Calories: 320 Fat: 10 g Carbohydrate: 15 g Protein: 45 g

MEAT

115. Tender Lamb Chops

Preparation Time: 10 minutes
Cooking Time: 6 hours
Servings: 8
INGREDIENTS:

- 8 lamb chops
- ½ teaspoon dried thyme
- 1 onion, sliced
- 1 teaspoon dried oregano
- 2 garlic cloves, minced
- Pepper and salt

DIRECTIONS:

1. Add sliced onion into the slow cooker.
2. Combine together thyme, oregano, pepper, and salt. Rub over lamb chops.
3. Place lamb chops in slow cooker and top with garlic.
4. Pour ¼ cup water around the lamb chops.
5. Cover and cook on low heat for 6 hours.
6. Serve and enjoy.

NUTRITION: Calories: 40 Fat: 1.9 g Carbohydrates: 2.3 g Sugar: 0.6 g Protein: 3.4 g Cholesterol: 0 mg

116. Smoky Pork & Cabbage

Preparation Time: 10 minutes
Cooking Time: 8 hours
Servings: 6
INGREDIENTS:

- 3 lbs pork roast
- 1/2 cabbage head, chopped
- 1 cup water
- 1/3 cup liquid smoke
- 1 tablespoon kosher salt

DIRECTIONS:

1. Rub pork with kosher salt and place into the crock pot.
2. Pour liquid smoke over the pork. Add water.
3. Cover and cook on low heat for 7 hours.
4. Remove pork from crock pot and add cabbage in the bottom of crock pot.
5. Place pork on top of the cabbage.
6. Cover again and cook for 1 more hour.
7. Shred pork with a fork and serve.

NUTRITION: Calories: 484 Fat: 21.5 g Carbohydrates: 4 g Sugar: 1.9 g Protein: 66 g Cholesterol: 195 mg

117. Seasoned Pork Chops

Preparation Time: 10 minutes
Cooking Time: 4 hours
Servings: 4
INGREDIENTS:

- 4 pork chops
- 2 garlic cloves, minced
- 1 cup chicken broth
- 1 tablespoon poultry seasoning
- 1/4 cup olive oil
- Pepper and salt

DIRECTIONS:

1. In a bowl, whisk together olive oil, poultry seasoning, garlic, broth, pepper, and salt.
2. Pour olive oil mixture into the slow cooker then place pork chops to the crock pot.
3. Cover and cook on high heat for 4 hours.
4. Serve and enjoy.

NUTRITION: Calories: 386 Fat: 32.9 g Carbohydrates: 3 g Sugar: 1 g Protein: 20 g Cholesterol: 70 mg

118. Beef Stroganoff

Preparation Time: 10 minutes
Cooking Time: 8 hours
Servings: 2
INGREDIENTS:

- 1/2 lb beef stew meat
- 10 oz mushroom soup, homemade
- 1 medium onion, chopped
- 1/2 cup sour cream
- 2.5 oz mushrooms, sliced
- Pepper and salt

DIRECTIONS:

1. Add all ingredients except sour cream into the crock pot and mix well.
2. Cover and cook on low heat for 8 hours.
3. Add sour cream and stir well.
4. Serve and enjoy.

NUTRITION: Calories 470 Fat 25 g Carbohydrates 8.6 g Sugar 3 g Protein 49 g Cholesterol 108 mg

119. Lemon Beef

Preparation Time: 10 minutes
Cooking Time: 6 hours
Servings: 4
INGREDIENTS:

- 1 lb beef chuck roast
- 1 fresh lime juice
- 1 garlic clove, crushed
- 1 teaspoon chili powder
- 2 cups lemon-lime soda
- 1/2 teaspoon salt

DIRECTIONS:

1. Place beef chuck roast into the slow cooker.
2. Season roast with garlic, chili powder, and salt.
3. Pour lemon-lime soda over the roast.
4. Cover slow cooker and cook on low for 6 hours. Shred the meat using fork.
5. Add lime juice over shredded roast and serve.

NUTRITION: Calories: 355 Fat: 16.8 g Carbohydrates: 14 g Sugar 11.3: g Protein 35.5: g Cholesterol: 120 mg

120. Herb Pork Roast

Preparation Time: 10 minutes
Cooking Time: 14 hours
Servings: 10
INGREDIENTS:

- 5 lbs pork roast, boneless or bone-in
- 1 tablespoon dry herb mix
- 4 garlic cloves, cut into slivers
- 1 tablespoon salt

DIRECTIONS:

1. Using a knife make small cuts all over meat then insert garlic slivers into the cuts.
2. In a small bowl, mix together Italian herb mix and salt and rub all over pork roast.
3. Place pork roast in the crock pot.
4. Cover and cook on low heat for 14 hours.
5. Extract meat from crock pot and shred using a fork.
6. Serve and enjoy.

NUTRITION: Calories: 327 Fat: 8 g Carbohydrates: 0.5 g Sugar: 0 g Protein: 59 g Cholesterol: 166 mg

121. Greek Beef Roast

Preparation Time: 10 minutes
Cooking Time: 8 hours
Servings: 6
INGREDIENTS:

- 2 lbs lean top round beef roast
- 1 tablespoon Italian seasoning
- 6 garlic cloves, minced
- 1 onion, sliced
- 2 cups beef broth
- ½ cup red wine
- 1 teaspoon red pepper flakes
- Pepper
- Salt

DIRECTIONS:

1. Season meat with pepper and salt and place into the crock pot.
2. Pour remaining ingredients over meat.
3. Cover and cook on low heat for 8 hours.
4. Shred the meat using fork.
5. Serve and enjoy.

NUTRITION: Calories: 231 Fat: 6 g Carbohydrates: 4 g Sugar: 1.4 g Protein: 35 g Cholesterol: 75 mg

122. Tomato Pork Chops

Preparation Time: 10 minutes
Cooking Time: 6 hours
Servings: 4
INGREDIENTS:

- 4 pork chops, bone-in
- 1 tablespoon garlic, minced
- ½ small onion, chopped
- 6 oz can tomato paste
- 1 bell pepper, chopped
- ¼ teaspoon red pepper flakes
- 1 teaspoon Worcestershire sauce
- 1 tablespoon dried Italian seasoning
  - oz can tomatoes, diced
- 2 teaspoon olive oil
- ¼ teaspoon pepper
- 1 teaspoon kosher salt

DIRECTIONS:

1. Heat oil in a pan over heat.
2. Season pork chops with pepper and salt.
3. Sear pork chops in pan until brown from both the sides.
4. Transfer pork chops into the crock pot.
5. Add remaining ingredients over pork chops.
6. Cover and cook on low heat for 6 hours.
7. Serve and enjoy.

NUTRITION: Calories: 325 Fat: 23.4 g Carbohydrates: 10 g Sugar: 6 g Protein: 20 g Cholesterol: 70 mg

123. Greek Pork Chops

Preparation Time: 10 minutes
Cooking Time: 6 minutes
Servings: 8
INGREDIENTS:

- 8 pork chops, boneless
- 4 teaspoon dried oregano
- 2 tablespoon Worcestershire sauce
- 3 tablespoon fresh lemon juice
- ¼ cup olive oil
- 1 teaspoon ground mustard
- 2 teaspoon garlic powder
- 2 teaspoon onion powder
- Pepper
- Salt

DIRECTIONS:

1. Whisk together oil, garlic powder, onion powder, oregano, Worcestershire sauce, lemon juice, mustard, pepper, and salt.
2. Place pork chops in a dish then pour marinade over pork chops and coat well. Place in refrigerator overnight.
3. Preheat the grill.
4. Place pork chops on the grill and cook for 3-4 minutes on each side.
5. Serve and enjoy.

NUTRITION: Calories: 324 Fat: 26.5 g Carbohydrates: 2.5 g Sugar: 1.3 g Protein: 18 g Cholesterol: 69 mg

124. Pork Cacciatore

Preparation Time: 10 minutes
Cooking Time: 6 hours
Servings: 6
INGREDIENTS:

- 1 ½ lbs pork chops
- 1 teaspoon dried oregano
- 1 cup beef broth
- 3 tablespoon tomato paste
- 14 oz can tomatoes, diced
- 2 cups mushrooms, sliced
- 1 small onion, diced
- 1 garlic clove, minced
- 2 tablespoon olive oil
- ¼ teaspoon pepper
- ½ teaspoon salt

DIRECTIONS:

1. Heat oil in a pan over medium heat.
2. Add pork chops in pan and cook until brown on both the sides.
3. Transfer pork chops into the crock pot.
4. Pour remaining ingredients over the pork chops.
5. Cover and cook on low heat for 6 hours.
6. Serve and enjoy.

NUTRITION: Calories: 440 Fat: 33 g Carbohydrates: 6 g Sugar: 3 g Protein: 28 g Cholesterol: 97 mg

125. Pork with Tomato & Olives

Preparation Time: 10 minutes
Cooking Time: 30 minutes
Servings: 6
INGREDIENTS:

- 6 pork chops, boneless and cut into thick slices
- 1/8 teaspoon ground cinnamon
- 1/2 cup olives, pitted and sliced
- 8 oz can tomatoes, crushed
- 1/4 cup beef broth
- 2 garlic cloves, chopped
- 1 large onion, sliced
- 1 tablespoon olive oil

DIRECTIONS:

1. Heat olive oil in a pan over medium heat.
2. Place pork chops in a pan and cook until lightly brown and set aside.
3. Cook onion and garlic in the same pan over medium heat, until onion is softened.
4. Add broth and bring to boil over high heat.
5. Return pork to pan and stir in crushed tomatoes and remaining ingredients.
6. Cover and simmer for 20 minutes.
7. Serve and enjoy.

NUTRITION: Calories: 321 Fat: 23 g Carbohydrates: 7 g Sugar: 1 g Protein: 19 g Cholesterol: 70 mg

126. Pork Roast

Preparation Time: 10 minutes
Cooking Time: 1 hour 35 minutes
Servings: 6
INGREDIENTS:

- 3 lbs pork roast, boneless
- 1 cup water
- 1 onion, chopped
- 3 garlic cloves, chopped
- 1 tablespoon black pepper
- 1 rosemary sprig
- 2 fresh oregano sprigs
- 2 fresh thyme sprigs
- 1 tablespoon olive oil
- 1 tablespoon kosher salt

DIRECTIONS:

1. Preheat the oven to 350 F.
2. Season pork roast with pepper and salt.
3. Heat olive oil in a stockpot and sear pork roast on each side, about 4 minutes.
4. Add onion and garlic. Pour in the water, oregano, and thyme and bring to boil for a minute.
5. Cover pot and roast in the preheated oven for 1 1/2 hours.
6. Serve and enjoy.

NUTRITION: Calories: 502 Fat: 23.8 g Carbohydrates: 3 g Sugar: 0.8 g Protein: 65 g Cholesterol: 195 mg

127. Easy Beef Kofta

Preparation Time: 10 minutes
Cooking Time: 10 minutes
Servings: 8
INGREDIENTS:

- 2 lbs ground beef
- 4 garlic cloves, minced
- 1 onion, minced
- 2 teaspoon cumin
- 1 cup fresh parsley, chopped
- ¼ teaspoon pepper
- 1 teaspoon salt

DIRECTIONS:

1. Add all the listed ingredients into the mixing bowl and mix until combined.
2. Roll meat mixture into the kabab shapes and cook in a hot pan for 4-6 minutes on each side or until cooked.
3. Serve and enjoy.

NUTRITION: Calories: 223 Fat: 7.3 g Carbohydrates: 2.5 g Sugar: 0.7 g Protein: 35 g Cholesterol: 101 mg

128. Lemon Pepper Pork Tenderloin

Preparation Time: 10 minutes
Cooking Time: 25 minutes
Servings: 4
INGREDIENTS:

- 1 lb pork tenderloin
- 3/4 teaspoon lemon pepper
- 2 teaspoon dried oregano
- 1 tablespoon olive oil
- 3 tablespoon feta cheese, crumbled
- 3 tablespoon olive tapenade

DIRECTIONS:

1. Add pork, oil, lemon pepper, and oregano in a zip-lock bag and rub well and place in a refrigerator for 2 hours.
2. Remove pork from zip-lock bag. Using sharp knife make lengthwise cut through the center of the tenderloin.
3. Spread olive tapenade on half tenderloin and sprinkle with feta cheese.
4. Fold another half of meat over to the original shape of tenderloin.
5. Tie close pork tenderloin with twine at 2-inch intervals.
6. Grill pork tenderloin for 20 minutes.
7. Cut into slices and serve.

NUTRITION: Calories: 215 Fat: 9.1 g Carbohydrates: 1 g Sugar: 0.5 g Protein: 30.8 g Cholesterol: 89 mg

VEGETABLES

129. Green Beans

Preparation time: 5 minutes
Cooking time: 13 minutes
Servings: 4
INGREDIENTS:

- 1-pound green beans
- ¾-teaspoon garlic powder
- ¾-teaspoon ground black pepper
- 1 ¼-teaspoon salt
- ½-teaspoon paprika

DIRECTIONS:

1. Switch on the air fryer, insert fryer basket, grease it with olive oil, then shut with its lid, set the fryer at 400 degrees F and preheat for 5 minutes.
2. Meanwhile, place beans in a bowl, spray generously with olive oil, sprinkle with garlic powder, black pepper, salt, and paprika and toss until well coated.
3. Open the fryer, add green beans in it, close with its lid and cook for 8 minutes until nicely golden and crispy, shaking halfway through the frying.
4. When air fryer beeps, open its lid, transfer green beans onto a serving plate and serve.

NUTRITION: Calories: 45 Carbs: 2 g Fat: 11 g Protein: 4 g Fiber: 3 g

130. Asparagus Avocado Soup

Preparation time: 10 minutes
Cooking time: 20 minutes
Servings: 4
INGREDIENTS:

- 1 avocado, peeled, pitted, cubed
- 12 ounces' asparagus
- ½-teaspoon ground black pepper
- 1-teaspoon garlic powder
- 1-teaspoon sea salt
- 2 tablespoons olive oil, divided
- 1/2 of a lemon, juiced
- 2 cups vegetable stock

DIRECTIONS:

1. Switch on the air fryer, insert fryer basket, grease it with olive oil, then shut with its lid, set the fryer at 425 degrees F and preheat for 5 minutes.
2. Meanwhile, place asparagus in a shallow dish, drizzle with 1-tablespoon oil, sprinkle with garlic powder, salt, and black pepper and toss until well mixed.
3. Open the fryer, add asparagus in it, close with its lid and cook for 10 minutes until nicely golden and roasted, shaking halfway through the frying.
4. When air fryer beeps, open its lid and transfer asparagus to a food processor.
5. Add remaining ingredients into a food processor and pulse until well combined and smooth.
6. Tip the soup in a saucepan, pour in water if the soup is too thick and heat it over medium-low heat for 5 minutes until thoroughly heated.
7. Ladle soup into bowls and serve.

NUTRITION: Calories: 208 Carbs: 2 g Fat: 11 g Protein: 4 g Fiber: 5 g

131. Sweet Potato Chips

Preparation time: 5 minutes
Cooking time: 10 minutes
Servings: 4
INGREDIENTS:

- 2 large sweet potatoes, cut into strips 25 mm thick
- 15 ml of oil
- 10g of salt
- 2g black pepper
- 2g of paprika
- 2g garlic powder
- 2g onion powder

DIRECTIONS:

1. Cut the sweet potatoes into strips 25 mm thick.
2. Preheat the air fryer for a few minutes.
3. Add the cut sweet potatoes in a large bowl and mix with the oil until the potatoes are all evenly coated.
4. Sprinkle salt, black pepper, paprika, garlic powder and onion powder. Mix well.
5. Place the French fries in the preheated baskets and cook for 10 minutes at 205°C (400°F). Be sure to shake the baskets halfway through cooking.

NUTRITION: Calories: 123 Carbs: 2 g Fat: 11 g Protein: 4 g Fiber: 0 g

132. Fried Zucchini

Preparation time: 10 minutes
Cooking time: 8 minutes
Servings: 4
INGREDIENTS:

- 2 medium zucchinis, cut into strips 19 mm thick
- 60g all-purpose flour
- 12g of salt
- 2g black pepper
- 2 beaten eggs
- 15 ml of milk
- 84g Italian seasoned breadcrumbs
- 25g grated Parmesan cheese
- Nonstick Spray Oil
- Ranch sauce, to serve

DIRECTIONS:

1. Cut the zucchini into strips 19 mm thick.
2. Mix with the flour, salt, and pepper on a plate. Mix the eggs and milk in a separate dish. Put breadcrumbs and Parmesan cheese in another dish.
3. Cover each piece of zucchini with flour, then dip them in egg and pass them through the crumbs. Leave aside.
4. Preheat the air fryer, set it to 175°C (345°F).
5. Place the covered zucchini in the preheated air fryer and spray with oil spray. Set the timer to 8 minutes and press Start / Pause.
6. Be sure to shake the baskets in the middle of cooking.
7. Serve with tomato sauce or ranch sauce.

NUTRITION: Calories: 68 Carbs: 2 g Fat: 11 g Protein: 4 g Fiber: 143g

133. Fried Avocado

Preparation time: 15 minutes
Cooking time: 10 minutes
Servings: 2
INGREDIENTS:

- 2 avocados cut into wedges 25 mm thick
- 50g Pan crumbs bread
- 2g garlic powder
- 2g onion powder
- 1g smoked paprika
- 1g cayenne pepper
- Salt and pepper to taste
- 60g all-purpose flour
- 2 eggs, beaten
- Nonstick Spray Oil
- Tomato sauce or ranch sauce, to serve

DIRECTIONS:

1. Cut the avocados into 25 mm thick pieces.
2. Combine the crumbs, garlic powder, onion powder, smoked paprika, cayenne pepper and salt in a bowl.
3. Separate each wedge of avocado in the flour, then dip the beaten eggs and stir in the breadcrumb mixture.
4. Preheat the air fryer.
5. Place the avocados in the preheated air fryer baskets, spray with oil spray and cook at 205°C (400°F) for 10 minutes. Turn the fried avocado halfway through cooking and sprinkle with cooking oil.
6. Serve with tomato sauce or ranch sauce.

NUTRITION: Calories: 123 Carbs: 2 g Fat: 11 g Protein: 4 g Fiber: 0 g

134. Vegetables in air Fryer

Preparation time: 20 minutes
Cooking time: 30 minutes
Servings: 2
INGREDIENTS:

- 2 potatoes
- 1 zucchini
- 1 onion
- 1 red pepper
- 1 green pepper

DIRECTIONS:

1. Cut the potatoes into slices.
2. Cut the onion into rings.
3. Cut the zucchini slices
4. Cut the peppers into strips.
5. Put all the ingredients in the bowl and add a little salt, ground pepper and some extra virgin olive oil.
6. Mix well.
7. Pass to the basket of the air fryer.
8. Select 160°C (320°F), 30 minutes.
9. Check that the vegetables are to your liking.

Nutrition: Calories: 135 Carbs: 2 g Fat: 11 g Protein: 4 g Fiber: 05g

135. Crispy Rye Bread Snacks with Guacamole and Anchovies

Preparation time: 10 minutes
Cooking time: 10 minutes
Servings: 4
INGREDIENTS:

- 4 slices of rye bread
- Guacamole
- Anchovies in oil

DIRECTIONS:

1. Cut each slice of bread into 3 strips of bread.
2. Place in the basket of the air fryer, without piling up, and we go in batches giving it the touch you want to give it. You can select 180°C (350°F), 10 minutes.
3. When you have all the crusty rye bread strips, put a layer of guacamole on top, whether homemade or commercial.
4. In each bread, place 2 anchovies on the guacamole.

NUTRITION: Calories: 180 Carbs: 4 g Fat: 11 g Protein: 4 g Fiber: 09 g

136. Mushrooms Stuffed with Tomato

Preparation time: 5 minutes
Cooking time: 50 minutes
Servings: 4
INGREDIENTS:

- 8 large mushrooms
- 250g of minced meat
- 4 cloves of garlic
- Extra virgin olive oil
- Salt
- Ground pepper
- Flour, beaten egg and breadcrumbs
- Frying oil
- Fried Tomato Sauce

DIRECTIONS:

1. Remove the stem from the mushrooms and chop it. Peel the garlic and chop. Put some extra virgin olive oil in a pan and add the garlic and mushroom stems.
2. Sauté and add the minced meat. Sauté well until the meat is well cooked and season.
3. Fill the mushrooms with the minced meat.
4. Press well and take the freezer for 30 minutes.
5. Pass the mushrooms with flour, beaten egg and breadcrumbs. Beaten egg and breadcrumbs.
6. Place the mushrooms in the basket of the air fryer.
7. Select 20 minutes, 180°C (350°F).
8. Distribute the mushrooms once cooked in the dishes.
9. Heat the tomato sauce and cover the stuffed mushrooms.

NUTRITION: Calories: 160 Carbs: 2 g Fat: 11 g Protein: 4 g Fiber: 0 g

STARCHES AND GRAINS

137. Faro with Artichoke Hearts

Preparation Time: 10 minutes
Cooking Time: 40 minutes
Servings: 6
INGREDIENTS:

- 1 cup faro
- 1 bay leaf
- 1 fresh rosemary sprig
- 1 fresh thyme sprig
- 2 tablespoons extra-virgin olive oil
- 1 onion, chopped
- 2 cups frozen artichoke hearts, thawed and chopped
- 1 tablespoon Italian seasoning
- 3 garlic cloves, minced
- 2 cups unsalted vegetable broth
- Zest of 1 lemon
- ½ teaspoon sea salt
- ¼ cup (about 2 ounces) grated Parmesan cheese

DIRECTIONS:

1. In a medium pot, combine the faro, bay leaf, rosemary, and thyme with enough water to cover it by about 2 inches. Place it on the stove top over medium-high heat and bring it to a boil. Reduce the heat to medium-low and simmer uncovered for 25 to 30 minutes, stirring occasionally, until the grain is tender. Drain any excess water and set the faro aside. Remove and discard the bay leaf, rosemary, and thyme.
2. In a large skillet over medium-high heat, heat the olive oil until it shimmers.
3. Add the onion, artichoke hearts, and Italian seasoning. Cook for about 5 minutes, stirring frequently, until the onion is soft.
4. Add the garlic and cook for 30 seconds, stirring constantly.
5. Add the broth, ½ cup at a time, and stir constantly until the liquid is absorbed before adding the next ½ cup of broth.
6. Stir in the lemon zest, sea salt, pepper, and cheese. Cook for 1 to 2 minutes more, stirring, until the cheese melts.

NUTRITION: Calories: 138 Protein: 7g Total Carbohydrates: 11g Sugars: 2g Fiber: 2g Total Fat: 8g Saturated Fat: 2g Cholesterol: 8mg Sodium: 522mg

138. Rice and Spinach

Preparation Time: 10 minutes
Cooking Time: 15 minutes
Servings: 6
INGREDIENTS:

- 2 tablespoons extra-virgin olive oil
- 1 onion, chopped
- 4 cups fresh baby spinach
- 1 garlic clove, minced
- Zest of 1 orange
- Juice of 1 orange
- 1 cup unsalted vegetable broth
- ½ teaspoon sea salt
- 2 cups cooked brown rice

DIRECTIONS:

1. In a large skillet over medium-high heat, heat the olive oil until it shimmers.
2. Add the onion and cook for about 5 minutes, stirring occasionally, until soft.
3. Add the spinach and cook for about 2 minutes, stirring occasionally, until it wilts.
4. Add the garlic and cook for 30 seconds, stirring constantly.
5. Stir in the orange zest and juice, broth, sea salt, and pepper. Bring to a simmer.
6. Stir in the rice and cook for about 4 minutes, stirring, until the rice is heated through and the liquid is absorbed.

NUTRITION: Calories: 188 Protein: 4g Total Carbohydrates: 31g Sugars: 4g Fiber: 3g Total Fat: 6g Saturated Fat: 1g Cholesterol: 0mg Sodium: 301mg

139. Spiced Couscous

Preparation Time: 10 minutes
Cooking Time: 15 minutes
Servings: 6
INGREDIENTS:

- 2 tablespoons extra-virgin olive oil
- ½ onion, minced
- Juice of 1 orange
- Zest of 1 orange
- ½ teaspoon garlic powder
- ½ teaspoon ground cumin
- ½ teaspoon sea salt
- ¼ teaspoon ground ginger
- ¼ teaspoon ground allspice
- ¼ teaspoon ground cinnamon
- 2 cups water
- 1 cup whole-wheat couscous
- ¼ cup dried apricots, chopped
- ¼ cup dried cranberries

DIRECTIONS:

1. In a medium saucepan over medium-high heat, heat the olive oil until it shimmers.
2. Add the onion and cook for about 3 minutes, stirring occasionally, until soft.
3. Add the orange juice and zest, garlic powder, cumin, sea salt, ginger, allspice, cinnamon, pepper, and water. Bring to a boil.
4. Add the couscous, apricots, and cranberries. Stir once, turn off the heat, and cover the pot. Let rest for 5 minutes, covered. Fluff with a fork.

NUTRITION: Calories: 181 Protein: 6g Total Carbohydrates: 30g Sugars: 5g Fiber: 4g Total Fat: 6g Saturated Fat: 1g Cholesterol: 0mg Sodium: 157mg

140. Sweet Potato Mash

Preparation Time: 10 minutes
Cooking Time: 20 minutes
Servings: 6
INGREDIENTS:

- 4 sweet potatoes, peeled and cubed
- ¼ cup almond milk
- ¼ cup extra-virgin olive oil
- ½ teaspoon sea salt

DIRECTIONS:

1. In a large pot over high heat, combine the sweet potatoes with enough water to cover by 2 inches. Bring the water to a boil. Reduce the heat to medium and cover the pot. Cook for 15 to 20 minutes until the potatoes are soft.
2. Drain the potatoes and return them to the dry pot off the heat. Add the almond milk, olive oil, sea salt, and pepper. With a potato masher, mash until smooth.

NUTRITION: Calories: 243 Protein: 2g Total Carbohydrates: 35g Sugars: 5g Fiber: 5g Total Fat: 11g Saturated Fat: 3g Cholesterol: 0mg Sodium: 169mg

141. Tabbouleh

Preparation Time: 10 minutes
Cooking Time: 0 minutes
Servings: 6
INGREDIENTS:

- 2 cups cooked whole-wheat couscous, cooled completely (see tip)
- 12 cherry tomatoes, quartered
- 6 scallions, white and green parts, minced
- 1 cucumber, peeled and chopped
- ½ cup fresh Italian parsley leaves, chopped
- ½ cup fresh mint leaves, chopped
- Juice of 2 lemons
- ¼ cup extra-virgin olive oil
- ½ teaspoon sea salt
- ¼ teaspoon freshly ground black pepper

DIRECTIONS:

1. In a large bowl, combine the couscous, tomatoes, scallions, cucumber, parsley, and mint. Set aside.
2. In a small bowl, whisk the lemon juice, olive oil, sea salt, and pepper. Toss with the couscous mixture. Let sit for 1 hour before serving.

NUTRITION: Calories: 254 Protein: 8g Total Carbohydrates: 38g Sugars: 9g Fiber: 7g Total Fat: 10g Saturated Fat: 2g Cholesterol: 0mg Sodium: 181mg

142. Orzo with Spinach and Feta

Preparation Time: 25 minutes
Cooking Time: 0 minutes
Servings: 6
INGREDIENTS:

- 6 cups fresh baby spinach, chopped
- ¼ cup scallions, white and green parts, chopped
- 1 (16-ounce) package orzo pasta, cooked according to package directions, rinsed, drained, and cooled
- ¾ cup crumbled feta cheese
- ¼ cup halved Kalamata olives
- ½ cup red wine vinegar
- ¼ cup extra-virgin olive oil
- 1½ teaspoons freshly squeezed lemon juice
- Sea salt
- Freshly ground black pepper

DIRECTIONS:

1. In a large bowl, combine the spinach, scallions, and cooled orzo.
2. Sprinkle with the feta and olives.
3. In a small bowl, whisk the vinegar, olive oil, and lemon juice. Season with sea salt and pepper.
4. Add the dressing to the salad and gently toss to combine. Refrigerate until serving.

NUTRITION: Calories: 255 Protein: 8g Total Carbohydrates: 38g Sugars: 3g Fiber: 2g Total Fat: 8g Saturated Fat: 2g Cholesterol: 5mg Sodium: 279mg

143. Pasta Puttanesca

Preparation Time: 10 minutes
Cooking Time: 10 minutes
INGREDIENTS:

- 2 tablespoons extra-virgin olive oil
- 6 garlic cloves, finely minced (or put through a garlic press)
- 2 teaspoons anchovy paste
- ¼ teaspoon red pepper flakes, plus more as needed
- 20 black olives, pitted and chopped
- 3 tablespoons capers, drained and rinsed
- ¼ teaspoon sea salt
- ¼ teaspoon freshly ground black pepper
- 2 (14-ounce) cans crushed tomatoes, undrained
- 1 (14-ounce) can chopped tomatoes, drained
- ¼ cup chopped fresh basil leaves
- 8 ounces' whole-wheat spaghetti, cooked according to package rinsed and drained

DIRECTIONS:

1. In a sauté pan or skillet over medium heat, stir together the olive oil, garlic, anchovy paste, and red pepper flakes. Cook for about 2 minutes, stirring, until the mixture is very fragrant.
2. Add the olives, capers, sea salt, and pepper.
3. In a blender, purée the crushed and chopped tomatoes and add to the pan. Cook for about 5 minutes, stirring occasionally, until the mixture simmers.
4. Stir in the basil and cooked pasta. Toss to coat the pasta with the sauce and serve.

NUTRITION: Calories: 278 Protein: 10g Total Carbohydrates: 40g Sugars: 16g Fiber: 12g Total Fat: 13g Saturated Fat: 1g Cholesterol: 9mg Sodium: 1,099mg

144. Pasta with Pesto

Preparation Time: 10 minutes
Cooking Time: 0 minutes
Servings: 4
INGREDIENTS:

- 3 tablespoons extra-virgin olive oil
- 3 garlic cloves, finely minced
- ½ cup fresh basil leaves
- ¼ cup (about 2 ounces) grated Parmesan cheese
- ¼ cup pine nuts
- 8 ounces' whole-wheat pasta, cooked according to package drained

DIRECTIONS:

1. In a blender or food processor, combine the olive oil, garlic, basil, cheese, and pine nuts. Pulse for 10 to 20 (1-second) pulses until everything is chopped and blended.
2. Toss with the hot pasta and serve.

NUTRITION: Calories: 405 Protein: 13g Total Carbohydrates: 44g Sugars: 2g Fiber: 5g Total Fat: 21g Saturated Fat: 4g Cholesterol: 10mg Sodium: 141mg

145. Sun-Dried Tomato and Artichoke Pizza

Preparation Time: 30 minutes
Cooking Time: 25 minutes
Servings: 6
INGREDIENTS:

- ¾ cup whole-wheat flour, plus more for flouring the work surface
- ¾ cup all-purpose flour
- 1 package quick-rising yeast
- ¾ teaspoon sea salt
- 2 tablespoons extra-virgin olive oil
- ¼ teaspoon honey
- Nonstick cooking spray
- For The Sauce:
- 2 tablespoons extra-virgin olive oil
- ½ onion, minced
- 3 garlic cloves, minced
- 1 (14-ounce) can crushed tomatoes
- 1 tablespoon dried oregano
- For The Pizza:
- 1 cup oil-packed sun-dried tomatoes, rinsed
- 2 cups frozen artichoke hearts
- ¼ cup (about 2 ounces) grated Asiago cheese

DIRECTIONS:

1. In a medium bowl, whisk the whole-wheat and all-purpose flours, yeast, and salt.
2. In a small bowl, whisk the hot water, olive oil, and honey.
3. Mix the liquids into the flour mixture and stir until sticky ball forms.
4. Turn the dough out onto a floured surface and knead for 5 minutes.
5. Coat a sheet of plastic wrap with cooking spray and cover the dough. Let rest for 10 minutes.
6. Roll the dough into a 13-inch circle.
7. In a saucepan over medium-high heat, heat the olive oil until it shimmers.
8. Add the onion and cook for 5 minutes, stirring occasionally.
9. Add the garlic and cook for 30 seconds, stirring constantly.
10. Stir in the tomatoes and oregano. Bring to a simmer. Reduce the heat to medium-low and simmer for 5 minutes more.
11. Preheat the oven to 500°F (or the hottest setting).
12. If you have a pizza stone, place it in the oven as it preheats.
13. In a thin layer, spread the sauce over the rolled dough.
14. Top the sauce with the artichoke hearts and sun-dried tomatoes. Sprinkle the cheese lightly over the top.
15. Place the pizza on the stone (or directly on the rack) and bake for 10 to 15 minutes until the crust is golden.

NUTRITION: Calories: 318 Protein: 12g Total Carbohydrates: 39g Sugars: 5g Fiber: 6g Total Fat: 14g Saturated Fat: 3g Cholesterol: 7mg Sodium: 524mg

FAST AND CHEAP

146. Creamed Coconut Curry Spinach

Preparation Time: 30 minutes
Cooking Time: 30 seconds
Servings: 6
INGREDIENTS:

- 1-pound frozen spinach, thawed and drained of moisture
- 1 small can whole fat coconut milk
- 2 teaspoons yellow curry paste
- 1 teaspoon lemon zest
- Cashews for garnish

DIRECTIONS:

1. Heat a medium sized pan to medium high heat, then add the curry paste and cook for 30 seconds. Add a small amount of the coconut milk and stir to combine, and then cook until the paste is aromatic.
2. Add the spinach, and then season. Separate the rest of the ingredients, from the cashews, and allow the sauce to reduce slightly.
3. Keep the sauce creamy, but reduce it to coat the spinach well. Serve with chopped cashews.

NUTRITION: Calories: 191 Total Carbohydrate: 9 g Cholesterol: 2 mg Total Fat: 14 g Fiber: 1 g Protein: 4 g

147. Shrimp Salad Cocktails

Preparation Time: 35 minutes
Cooking Time: 35 minutes
Servings: 8 servings
INGREDIENTS:

- 2 cups mayonnaise
- 6 plum tomatoes, seeded and finely chopped
- 1/4 cup ketchup
- 1/4 cup lemon juice
- 2 cups seedless red and/or green grapes, halved
- 1 tablespoon. Worcestershire sauce
- 2 lbs. peeled and deveined cooked large shrimp
- 2 celery ribs, finely chopped
- 3 tablespoons. minced fresh tarragon or 3 teaspoon dried tarragon
- salt and 1/4 teaspoon pepper
- shredded 2 of cups romaine
- papaya or 1/2 cup peeled chopped mango
- parsley or minced chives

DIRECTIONS:

1. Combine Worcestershire sauce, lemon juice, ketchup and mayonnaise together in a small bowl. Combine pepper, salt, tarragon, celery and shrimp together in a large bowl. Put in 1 cup of dressing toss well to coat.
2. Scoop 1 tablespoon. of the dressing into 8 cocktail glasses. Layer each glass with 1/4 cup of lettuce, followed by 1/2 cup of the shrimp mixture, 1/4 cup of grapes, 1/3 cup of tomatoes and finally 1 tablespoon. of mango. Spread the remaining dressing over top; sprinkle chives on top. Serve immediately.

NUTRITION: Calories: 580 Total Carbohydrate: 16 g Cholesterol: 192 mg Total Fat: 46 g Fiber: 2 g Protein: 24 g

148. Garlic Chive Cauliflower Mash

Preparation Time: 20 minutes
Cooking Time: 18 minutes
Servings: 5
INGREDIENTS:

- 4 cups cauliflower
- 1/3 cup vegetarian mayonnaise
- 1 garlic clove
- 1/2 teaspoon. kosher salt
- 1 tablespoon. water
- 1/8 teaspoon. pepper
- 1/4 teaspoon. lemon juice
- 1/2 teaspoon lemon zest
- 1 tablespoon Chives, minced

DIRECTIONS:

1. In a bowl that is save to microwave, add the cauliflower, mayo, garlic, water, and salt/pepper and mix until the cauliflower is well coated. Cook on high for 15-18 minutes, until the cauliflower is almost mushy.
2. Blend the mixture in a strong blender until completely smooth, adding a little more water if the mixture is too chunky. Season with the remaining ingredients and serve.

NUTRITION: Calories: 178 Total Carbohydrate: 14 g Cholesterol: 18 mg Total Fat: 18 g Fiber: 4 g Protein: 2 g

149. Beet Greens with Pine Nuts Goat Cheese

Preparation Time: 25 minutes
Cooking Time: 15 minutes
Servings: 3
INGREDIENTS:

- 4 cups beet tops, washed and chopped roughly
- 1 teaspoon. EVOO
- 1 tablespoon. no sugar added balsamic vinegar
- 2 oz. crumbled dry goat cheese
- 2 tablespoons. Toasted pine nuts

DIRECTIONS:

1. Warm the oil in a pan, then cook the beet greens on medium high heat until they release their moisture. Let it cook until almost tender. Flavor with salt and pepper and remove from heat.
2. Toss the greens in a mixture of balsamic vinegar and olive oil, then top with the nuts and cheese. Serve warm.

NUTRITION: Calories: 215 Total Carbohydrate: 4 g Cholesterol: 12 mg Total Fat: 18 g Fiber: 2 g Protein: 10 g

150. Shrimp with Dipping Sauce

Preparation Time: 5 minutes
Cooking Time: 15 minutes
Servings: 6
INGREDIENTS:

- 1 tablespoon. reduced-sodium soy sauce
- 2 teaspoons. Hot pepper sauce
- 1 teaspoon. canola oil
- 1/4 teaspoon. garlic powder
- 1/8 to 1/4 teaspoon. cayenne pepper
- 1 lb. uncooked medium shrimp, peeled and deveined
- 2 tablespoons. Chopped green onions
- Dipping Sauce:
- 3 tablespoons Reduced-sodium soy sauce
- 1 teaspoon. rice vinegar
- 1 tablespoon. orange juice
- 2 teaspoons. Sesame oil
- 2 teaspoons. Honey
- 1 garlic clove, minced
- 1-1/2 teaspoons. Minced fresh gingerroot

DIRECTIONS:

1. Heat the initial 5 ingredients in a big nonstick frying pan for 30 seconds, then mix continuously. Add onions and shrimp and stir fry for 4-5 minutes or until the shrimp turns pink. Mix together the sauce and serve it with the shrimp.

NUTRITION: Calories: 97 Total Carbohydrate: 4 g Cholesterol: 112 mg Total Fat: 3 g Fiber: 0 g Protein: 13 g

151. Celeriac Cauliflower Mash

Preparation Time: 20 minutes
Cooking Time: 12 minutes
Servings: 6
INGREDIENTS:

- 1 head cauliflower
- 1 small celery root
- 1/4 cup butter
- 1 tablespoon. chopped rosemary
- 1 tablespoon. chopped thyme
- 1 cup cream cheese

DIRECTIONS:

1. Skin the celery root and cut into small pieces. Cut the cauliflower into similar sized pieces and combine.
2. Toast the herbs in the butter in a large pan, until they become fragrant. Add the cauliflower and celery root and stir to combine. Season and cook at medium high until whatever moisture is in the vegetables releases itself, then covers and cook on low for 10-12 minutes.
3. Once the vegetables are soft, remove from the heat and place them in the blender. Make it smooth, then put the cream cheese and puree again. Season and serve.

NUTRITION: Calories: 225 Total Carbohydrate: 4 g Cholesterol: 1 mg Total Fat: 20 g Fiber: 0 g Protein: 5 g

152. Cheddar Drop Biscuits

Easy/Diary-free
Preparation Time: 30 minutes
Cooking Time: 15 minutes
Servings: 8
INGREDIENTS:

- 1/4 cup coconut oil
- 4 eggs
- 2 teaspoon apple cider vinegar
- 1 1/2 cup coarse almond meal
- 1/2 teaspoon. baking powder, gluten free
- 1/2 teaspoon. onion powder
- 1/4 teaspoon. salt
- 3/4 cup cheddar cheese
- 2 tablespoons. Chopped jalapenos

DIRECTIONS:

1. Line a sheet tray with parchment paper, and then preheat the oven to 400F
2. Mix the wet ingredients in a bowl until combined, then reserve. Mix the dry ingredients in a separate bowl until combined, and then add them to the wet ingredients, stirring until incorporated. Fold in the cheddar cheese and jalapenos.
3. Drop the dough onto the parchment paper into eight roughly equal pieces, and then shape as desired once they are on the tray.
4. Bake until golden brown, 12-15 minutes. Rotate the tray halfway through baking so browning is even.
5. Cool slightly and serve.

NUTRITION: Calories: 260 Total Carbohydrate: 4 g Cholesterol: 8 mg Total Fat: 22 g Fiber: 1 g Protein: 4 g

153. Roasted Radish with Fresh Herbs

Preparation Time: 15 minutes
Cooking Time: 10 minutes
Servings: 4
INGREDIENTS:

- 1 tablespoon. coconut oil
- 1 bunch radishes
- 2 tablespoons. Minced chives
- 1 tablespoon. minced rosemary
- 1 tablespoon. minced thyme

DIRECTIONS:

1. Wash the radishes, and then remove the tops and stems. Cut them into quarters and reserve.
2. Add the oil to a cast iron pan, then heat to medium. Add the radishes, and then season with salt and pepper. Cook on medium heat for 6-8 minutes, until almost tender, then add the herbs and cook through.
3. The radishes can be served warm with meats or chilled with salads.

NUTRITION: Calories: 123 Total Carbohydrate: 6 g Cholesterol: 8 mg Total Fat: 13 g Fiber: 2 g Protein: 6 g

154. Tomato Cheddar Fondue

Preparation Time: 20 minutes
Cooking Time: 30 minutes
Servings: 3-1/2 cups
INGREDIENTS:

- 1 garlic clove, halved
- 6 medium tomatoes, seeded and diced
- 2/3 cup dry white wine
- 6 tablespoons. Butter, cubed
- 1-1/2 teaspoons. Dried basil
- Dash cayenne pepper
- 2 cups shredded cheddar cheese
- 1 tablespoon. All-purpose flour
- Cubed French bread and cooked shrimp

DIRECTIONS:

1. Rub the bottom and sides of a fondue pot with a garlic clove. Set aside and discard the garlic.
2. Combine wine, butter, basil, cayenne and tomatoes in a large saucepan. On a medium low heat, bring mixture to a simmer, then decrease heat to low. Mix cheese with flour. Add to tomato mixture gradually while stirring after each addition until cheese is melted.
3. Pour into the Preparation timeared fondue pot and keep warm. Enjoy with shrimp and bread cubes.

NUTRITION: Calories: 118 Total Carbohydrate: 4 g Cholesterol: 30 mg Total Fat: 10 g Fiber: 1 g Protein: 4 g

155. Swiss Seafood Canapés

Preparation Time: 20 minutes
Cooking Time: 25 minutes
Servings: 4 dozen.
INGREDIENTS:

- 1 can (6 oz.) small shrimp, rinsed and drained
- 1 package (6 oz.) frozen crabmeat, thawed
- 1 cup shredded Swiss cheese
- 2 hard-boiled large eggs, chopped
- 1/4 cup finely chopped celery
- 1/4 cup mayonnaise
- 1/4 cup French salad dressing or seafood cocktail sauce
- 2 green onions, chopped
- Dash salt
- 1 loaf (16 oz.) snack rye bread

DIRECTIONS:

1. Mix the first nine ingredients in a large bowl. Put bread on ungreased baking sheets. Broil for 1 to 2 minutes, 4 to 6-inches from the heat or until lightly browned. Flip slices over; spread 1 rounded tablespoonful of seafood mixture on each. Broil for 4 to 5 more minutes or until heated through.

NUTRITION: Calories: 57 Total Carbohydrate: 5 g Cholesterol: 22 mg Total Fat: 3 g Fiber: 1 g Protein: 3 g

156. Squash & Zucchini

Preparation Time: 5 min
Cooking Time: 4-6 hours
Servings: 6
INGREDIENTS:

- Zucchini (sliced and quartered) – 2 cups
- Yellow squash (sliced and quartered) – 2 cups
- Pepper – ¼ teaspoon
- Italian seasoning – 1 teaspoon
- Garlic powder – 1 teaspoon
- Sea salt – ½ teaspoon
- Butter (cubed) – ¼ cup
- Parmesan cheese (grated) – ¼ cup

DIRECTIONS:

1. Combine all the ingredients in the slow cooker.
2. Cook covered for 4-6 hours on low.

NUTRITION: Calories: 122 Total Carbohydrate: 4 g Cholesterol: 18 mg Total Fat: 9.9 g Fiber: 4 g Protein: 14 g

SOUP AND SALAD

157. Taste of Normandy Salad

Preparation Time:25 minutes
Cooking Time: 5 minutes
Servings:4 to 6
INGREDIENTS:

- For the walnuts
- 2 tablespoons butter
- ¼ cup sugar or honey
- 1 cup walnut pieces
- ½ teaspoon kosher salt
- For the dressing
- 3 tablespoons extra-virgin olive oil
- 1½ tablespoons champagne vinegar
- 1½ tablespoons Dijon mustard
- ¼ teaspoon kosher salt
- For the salad
- 1 head red leaf lettuce, shredded into pieces
- 3 heads endive, ends trimmed and leaves separated
- 2 apples, cored and divided into thin wedges
- 1 (8-ounce) Camembert wheel, cut into thin wedges

DIRECTION:

1. To make the walnuts
2. Dissolve the butter in a skillet over medium high heat. Stir in the sugar and cook until it dissolves. Add the walnuts and cook for about 5 minutes, stirring, until toasty. Season with salt and transfer to a plate to cool.
3. To make the dressing
4. Whip the oil, vinegar, mustard, and salt in a large bowl until combined.
5. To make the salad
6. Add the lettuce and endive to the bowl with the dressing and toss to coat. Transfer to a serving platter.
7. Decoratively arrange the apple and Camembert wedges over the lettuce and scatter the walnuts on top. Serve immediately.
8. Meal Prep Tip: Prepare the walnuts in advance—in fact, double the quantities and use them throughout the week to add a healthy crunch to salads, oats, or simply to enjoy as a snack.

NUTRITION: Calories: 699 Total fat: 52g Total carbs: 44g Cholesterol: 60mg Fiber: 17g Protein: 23g Sodium: 1170mg

158. Loaded Caesar Salad with Crunchy Chickpeas

Preparation Time:5 minutes
Cooking Time:20 minutes
Servings:6
INGREDIENT:

- For the chickpeas
- 2 (15-ounce) cans chickpeas, drained and rinsed
- 2 tablespoons extra-virgin olive oil
- 1 teaspoon kosher salt
- 1 teaspoon garlic powder
- 1 teaspoon onion powder
- 1 teaspoon dried oregano
- For the dressing
- ½ cup mayonnaise
- 2 tablespoons grated Parmesan cheese
- 2 tablespoons freshly squeezed lemon juice
- 1 clove garlic, peeled and smashed
- 1 teaspoon Dijon mustard
- ½ tablespoon Worcestershire sauce
- ½ tablespoon anchovy paste
- For the salad
- 3 heads romaine lettuce, cut into bite-size pieces

DIRECTION:

1. To make the chickpeas
2. Preheat the oven to 450°F. Line a baking sheet with parchment paper.
3. Add the chickpeas, oil, salt, garlic powder, onion powder, and oregano in a small container. Scatter the coated chickpeas on the prepared baking sheet.
4. Roast for about 20 minutes, tossing occasionally, until the chickpeas are golden and have a bit of crunch.
5. To make the dressing
6. In a small bowl, whisk the mayonnaise, Parmesan, lemon juice, garlic, mustard, Worcestershire sauce, and anchovy paste until combined.
7. To make the salad
8. Combine the lettuce and dressing in a large container. Toss to coat. Top with the roasted chickpeas and serve.
9. Cooking Tip: Don't wash out that bowl you used for the chickpeas—the remaining oil adds a great punch of flavor to blanched green beans or another simply cooked vegetable.

NUTRITION: Calories: 367 Total fat: 22g Total carbs: 35g Cholesterol: 9mg Fiber: 13g Protein: 12g Sodium: 407mg

159. Coleslaw worth a Second Helping

Preparation Time:20 minutes
Cooking Time:10 minutes
Servings:6
INGREDIENTS:

- 5 cups shredded cabbage
- 2 carrots, shredded
- ½ cup mayonnaise
- ½ cup sour cream
- 3 tablespoons apple cider vinegar
- 1 teaspoon kosher salt
- ½ teaspoon celery seed

DIRECTION:

1. Add together the cabbage, carrots, and parsley in a large bowl.
2. Whisk together the mayonnaise, sour cream, vinegar, salt, and celery in a small bowl until smooth. Pour sauce over veggies and pour until covered. Transfer to a serving bowl and bake until ready to serve.

NUTRITION: Calories: 192 Total fat: 18g Total carbs: 7g Cholesterol: 18mg Fiber: 3g Protein: 2g Sodium: 543mg

160. Romaine Lettuce and Radicchios Mix

Preparation Time:6 minutes
Cooking Time:0 minutes
Servings:4
INGREDIENTS:

- 2 tablespoons olive oil
- A pinch of salt and black pepper
- 2 spring onions, chopped
- 3 tablespoons Dijon mustard
- Juice of 1 lime
- ½ cup basil, chopped
- 4 cups romaine lettuce heads, chopped
- 3 radicchios, sliced

DIRECTIONS:

1. In a salad bowl, blend the lettuce with the spring onions and the other ingredients, toss and serve.

NUTRITION: Calories: 87 Fats: 2 g Fiber: 1 g Carbs: 1 g Protein: 2 g

161. Greek Salad

Preparation Time:15 Minutes
Cooking Time:15 Minutes
Servings:5
INGREDIENTS:

- For Dressing:
- ½ teaspoon black pepper
- ¼ teaspoon salt
- ½ teaspoon oregano
- 1 tablespoon garlic powder
- 2 tablespoons Balsamic
- 1/3 cup olive oil
- For Salad:
- ½ cup sliced black olives
- ½ cup chopped parsley, fresh
- 1 small red onion, thin-sliced
- 1 cup cherry tomatoes, sliced
- 1 bell pepper, yellow, chunked
- 1 cucumber, peeled, quarter and slice
- 4 cups chopped romaine lettuce
- ½ teaspoon salt
- 2 tablespoons olive oil

DIRECTIONS:

1. In a small container, join all of the ingredients for the dressing and let this set in the freezer while you make the salad.
2. To assemble the salad, mix together all the ingredients in a large-sized bowl and toss the veggies gently but thoroughly to mix.
3. Serve the salad with the dressing in amounts as desired

NUTRITION: Calories: 234 Fat: 16.1 g Protein: 5 g Carbs: 48 g

162. Asparagus and Smoked Salmon Salad

Preparation Time:15 minutes
Cooking Time:10 minutes
Servings:8
INGREDIENTS:

- 1 lb. fresh asparagus, shaped and cut into 1 inch pieces
- 1/2 cup pecans, smashed into pieces
- 2 heads red leaf lettuce, washed and split
- 1/2 cup frozen green peas, thawed
- 1/4 lb. smoked salmon, cut into 1 inch chunks
- 1/4 cup olive oil
- 2 tablespoons. lemon juice
- 1 teaspoon Dijon mustard
- 1/2 teaspoon salt
- 1/4 teaspoon pepper

DIRECTIONS:

1. Boil a pot of water. Stir in asparagus and cook for 5 minutes until tender. Let it drain; set aside.
2. In a skillet, cook the pecans over medium heat for 5 minutes, stirring constantly until lightly toasted.
3. Combine the asparagus, toasted pecans, salmon, peas, and red leaf lettuce and toss in a large bowl.
4. In another bowl, combine lemon juice, pepper, Dijon mustard, salt, and olive oil. You can coat the salad with the dressing or serve it on its side.

NUTRITION: Calories: 159 Total Carbohydrate: 7 g Cholesterol: 3 mg Total Fat: 12.9 g Protein: 6 g Sodium: 304 mg

163. Shrimp Cobb Salad

Preparation Time:25 minutes
Cooking Time:10 minutes
Servings: 2
INGREDIENTS:

- 4 slices center-cut bacon
- 1 lb. large shrimp, peeled and deveined
- 1/2 teaspoon ground paprika
- 1/4 teaspoon ground black pepper
- 1/4 teaspoon salt, divided
- 2 1/2 tablespoons. Fresh lemon juice
- 1 1/2 tablespoons. Extra-virgin olive oil
- 1/2 teaspoon whole grain Dijon mustard
- 1 (10 oz.) package romaine lettuce hearts, chopped
- 2 cups cherry tomatoes, quartered
- 1 ripe avocado, cut into wedges
- 1 cup shredded carrots

DIRECTIONS:

1. Cook the bacon for 4 minutes on each side in a large skillet over medium heat till crispy.
2. Take away from the skillet and place on paper towels; let cool for 5 minutes. Break the bacon into bits. Throw out most of the bacon fat, leaving behind only 1 tablespoon. in the skillet. Bring the skillet back to medium-high heat. Add black pepper and paprika to the shrimp for seasoning. Cook the shrimp around 2 minutes each side until it is opaque. Sprinkle with 1/8 teaspoon of salt for seasoning.
3. Combine the remaining 1/8 teaspoon of salt, mustard, olive oil and lemon juice together in a small bowl. Stir in the romaine hearts.
4. On each serving plate, place on 1 and 1/2 cups of romaine lettuce. Add on top the same amounts of avocado, carrots, tomatoes, shrimp and bacon.

NUTRITION: Calories: 528 Total Carbohydrate: 22.7 g Cholesterol: 365 mg Total Fat: 28.7 g Protein: 48.9 g Sodium: 1166 mg

164. Toast with Smoked Salmon, Herbed Cream Cheese, and Greens

Preparation Time:10 minutes
Cooking Time:5 minutes
Servings:2
INGREDIENTS:

- For the herbed cream cheese
- ¼ cup cream cheese, at room temperature
- 2 tablespoons chopped fresh flat-leaf parsley
- 2 tablespoons chopped fresh chives or sliced scallion
- ½ teaspoon garlic powder
- ¼ teaspoon kosher salt
- For the toast
- 2 slices bread
- 4 ounces smoked salmon
- Small handful microgreens or sprouts
- 1 tablespoon capers, drained and rinsed
- ¼ small red onion, very thinly sliced

DIRECTIONS:

1. To make the herbed cream cheese
2. In a small container, put together the cream cheese, parsley, chives, garlic powder, and salt. Using a fork, mix until combined. Chill until ready to use.
3. To make the toast
4. Toast the bread until golden. Spread the herbed cream cheese over each piece of toast, then top with the smoked salmon.
5. Garnish with the microgreens, capers, and red onion.

NUTRITION: Calories: 194 Total fat: 8g Cholesterol: 26mg Fiber: 2g Protein: 12g Sodium: 227mg

SMOOTHIES

165. Avocado Blueberry Smoothie

Preparation Time: 5 minutes
Cooking Time: 5 minutes
Servings: 1
INGREDIENTS:

- 1 tsp chia seeds
- ½ cup unsweetened coconut milk
- 1 avocado
- ½ cup blueberries

DIRECTIONS:

1. Add all the listed ingredients to the blender and blend until smooth and creamy.
2. Serve immediately and enjoy.

NUTRITION: Calories: 389 Fat: 34.6g Carbs: 20.7g Protein: 4.8g Fiber: 0g

166. Vegan Blueberry Smoothie

Preparation Time: 5 minutes
Cooking Time: 5 minutes
Servings: 2
INGREDIENTS:

- 2 cups blueberries
- 1 tbsp hemp seeds
- 1 tbsp chia seeds
- 1 tbsp flax meal
- 1/8 tsp orange zest, grated
- 1 cup fresh orange juice
- 1 cup unsweetened coconut milk

DIRECTIONS:

1. Toss all your ingredients into your blender then process till smooth and creamy.
2. Serve immediately and enjoy.

NUTRITION: Calories: 212 Fat: 6.6g Carbs: 36.9g Protein: 5.2g Fiber: 0g

167. Berry Peach Smoothie

Preparation Time: 5 minutes
Cooking Time: 5 minutes
Servings: 2
INGREDIENTS:

- 1 cup coconut water
- 1 tbsp hemp seeds
- 1 tbsp agave
- ½ cup strawberries
- ½ cup blueberries
- ½ cup cherries
- ½ cup peaches

DIRECTIONS:

1. Toss all your ingredients into your blender then process till smooth and creamy.
2. Serve immediately and enjoy.

NUTRITION: Calories: 117 Fat: 2.5g Carbs: 22.5g Protein: 3.5g Fiber: 0g

168. Cantaloupe Blackberry Smoothie

Preparation Time: 5 minutes
Cooking Time: 5 minutes
Servings: 2
INGREDIENTS:

- 1 cup coconut milk yogurt
- ½ cup blackberries
- 2 cups fresh cantaloupe
- 1 banana

DIRECTIONS:

1. Toss all your ingredients into your blender then process till smooth.
2. Serve and enjoy.

NUTRITION: Calories: 160 Fat: 4.5g Carbs: 33.7g Protein: 1.8g Fiber: 0g

169. Cantaloupe Kale Smoothie

Preparation Time: 5 minutes
Cooking Time: 5 minutes
Servings: 2
INGREDIENTS:

- 8 oz. water
- 1 orange, peeled
- 3 cups kale, chopped
- 1 banana, peeled
- 2 cups cantaloupe, chopped
- 1 zucchini, chopped

DIRECTIONS:

1. Toss all your ingredients into your blender then process till smooth and creamy.
2. Serve immediately and enjoy.

NUTRITION: Calories: 203 Fat: 0.5g Carbs: 49.2g Protein: 5.6g Fiber: 0g

170. Mix Berry Cantaloupe Smoothie

Preparation Time: 5 minutes
Cooking Time: 5 minutes
Servings: 2
INGREDIENTS:

- 1 cup alkaline water
- 2 fresh Seville orange juices
- ¼ cup fresh mint leaves
- 1 ½ cups mixed berries
- 2 cups cantaloupe

DIRECTIONS

1. Toss all your ingredients into your blender then process till smooth.
2. Serve immediately and enjoy.

NUTRITION: Calories: 122 Fat: 1g Carbs: 26.1g Protein: 2.4g Fiber: 0g

171. Avocado Kale Smoothie

Preparation Time: 5 minutes
Cooking Time: 5 minutes
Servings: 3
INGREDIENTS:

- 1 cup water
- ½ Seville orange, peeled
- 1 avocado
- 1 cucumber, peeled
- 1 cup kale
- 1 cup ice cubes

DIRECTIONS:

1. Toss all your ingredients into your blender then process till smooth and creamy.
2. Serve immediately and enjoy.

NUTRITION: Calories: 160 Fat: 13.3g Carbs: 11.6g Protein: 2.4g Fiber: 0g

172. Apple Kale Cucumber Smoothie

Preparation Time: 5 minutes
Cooking Time: 5 minutes
Servings: 1
INGREDIENTS:

- ¾ cup water
- ½ green apple, diced
- ¾ cup kale
- ½ cucumber

DIRECTIONS:

1. Toss all your ingredients into your blender then process till smooth and creamy.
2. Serve immediately and enjoy.

NUTRITION: Calories: 86 Fat: 0.5g Carbs: 21.7g Protein: 1.9g Fiber: 0g

173. Refreshing Cucumber Smoothie

Preparation Time: 5 minutes
Cooking Time: 5 minutes
Servings: 2
INGREDIENTS:

- 1 cup ice cubes
- 20 drops liquid stevia
- 2 fresh lime, peeled and halved
- 1 tsp lime zest, grated
- 1 cucumber, chopped
- 1 avocado, pitted and peeled
- 2 cups kale
- 1 tbsp creamed coconut
- ¾ cup coconut water

DIRECTIONS:

1. Toss all your ingredients into your blender then process till smooth and creamy.
2. Serve immediately and enjoy.

NUTRITION: Calories: 313 Fat: 25.1g Carbs: 24.7g Protein: 4.9g Fiber: 0g

174. Cauliflower Veggie Smoothie

Preparation Time: 5 minutes
Cooking Time: 5 minutes
Servings: 4
INGREDIENTS:

- 1 zucchini, peeled and chopped
- 1 Seville orange, peeled
- 1 apple, diced
- 1 banana
- 1 cup kale
- ½ cup cauliflower

DIRECTIONS:

1. Toss all your ingredients into your blender then process till smooth and creamy.
2. Serve immediately and enjoy.

NUTRITION: Calories: 71 Fat: 0.3g Carbs: 18.3g Protein: 1.3g Fiber: 0g

175. Soursop Smoothie

Preparation Time: 5 minutes
Cooking Time: 5 Minutes
Servings: 2
INGREDIENTS:

1. 3 quartered frozen Burro Bananas
2. 1-1/2 cups of Homemade Coconut Milk
3. 1/4 cup of Walnuts
4. 1 teaspoon of Sea Moss Gel
5. 1 teaspoon of Ground Ginger
6. 1 teaspoon of Soursop Leaf Powder
7. 1 handful of Kale

Directions:

1. Prepare and put all ingredients in a blender or a food processor.
2. Blend it well until you reach a smooth consistency.
3. Serve and enjoy your Soursop Smoothie!
4. Useful Tips:
5. If you don't have frozen Bananas, you can use fresh ones.

NUTRITION: Calories: 213 Fat: 3.1gCarbs: 6g Protein: 8g Fiber: 4.3g

176. Cucumber-Ginger Water

Preparation Time: 5 minutes
Cooking Time: 5 Minutes
Servings: 2
INGREDIENTS:

- 1 sliced Cucumber
- 1 smashed thumb of Ginger Root
- 2 cups of Spring Water

DIRECTIONS:

1. Prepare and put all ingredients in a jar with a lid.
2. Let the water infuse overnight. Store it in the refrigerator.
3. Serve and enjoy your Cucumber-Ginger Water throughout the day!

NUTRITION: Calories: 117 Fat: 2g Carbs: 6g Protein: 9.7g Fiber: 2g

177. Strawberry Milkshake

Preparation Time: 5 minutes
Cooking Time: 5 Minutes
Servings: 2
INGREDIENTS:

- 2 cups of Homemade Hempseed Milk
- 1 cup of frozen Strawberries
- Agave Syrup, to taste

DIRECTIONS:

1. Prepare and put all ingredients in a blender or a food processor.
2. Blend it well until you reach a smooth consistency.
3. Serve and enjoy your Strawberry Milkshake!
4. Useful Tips
5. If you don't have Homemade Hempseed Milk, you can add Homemade Walnut Milk instead.
6. If you don't have frozen Strawberries, you can use fresh ones.

NUTRITION: Calories: 222 Fat: 4g Carbs: 3g Protein: 6g Fiber: 1g

178. Cactus Smoothie

Preparation Time: 5 minutes
Cooking Time: 10 Minutes
Servings: 2
INGREDIENTS:

- 1 medium Cactus
- 2 cups of Homemade Coconut Milk
- 2 frozen Baby Bananas
- 1/2 cup of Walnuts
- 1 Date
- 2 teaspoons of Hemp Seeds

DIRECTIONS:

1. Take the Cactus, remove all pricks, wash it, and cut into medium pieces.
2. Put all the listed ingredients in a blender or a food processor.
3. Blend it well until you reach a smooth consistency.
4. Serve and enjoy your Cactus Smoothie!
5. Useful Tips
6. If you don't have Homemade Coconut Milk, you can add Homemade Walnut Milk or Homemade Hempseed Milk instead.
7. If you don't have frozen Bananas, you can use fresh ones.
8. If you don't have Baby Bananas, add 1 Burro Banana instead.

NUTRITION: Calories: 123 Fat: 3g Carbs: 6g Protein: 2.5g Fiber: 0g

179. Prickly Pear Juice

Preparation Time: 5 minutes
Cooking Time: 10 Minutes
Servings: 2
INGREDIENTS:

- 6 Prickly Pears
- 1/3 cup of Lime Juice
- 1/3 cup of Agave
- 1-1/2 cups of Spring Water*

DIRECTIONS:

1. Take Prickly Pear, cut off the ends, slice off the skin, and put in a blender. Do the same with the other pears.
2. Add Lime Juice with Agave to the blender and blend well for 30–40 seconds.
3. Strain the prepared mixture through a nut milk bag or cheesecloth and pour it back into the blender.
4. Pour Spring Water in and blend it repeatedly.
5. Serve and enjoy your Prickly Pear Juice!
6. Useful Tips:
7. If you want a cold drink, add a tray of ice cubes instead.
8. like and serve it on top of the braised greens.

NUTRITION: Calories: 312 Fat: 6g Carbs: 11g Protein: 8g Fiber: 2g

SNACKS

180. Veggie Fritters

Preparation Time: 10 minutes
Cooking Time: 10 minutes
Servings: 4
INGREDIENTS:

- 2 garlic cloves, minced
- 2 yellow onions, chopped
- 4 scallions, chopped
- 2 carrots, grated
- 2 teaspoons cumin, ground
- ½ teaspoon turmeric powder
- Salt and black pepper to the taste
- ¼ teaspoon coriander, ground
- 2 tablespoons parsley, chopped
- ¼ teaspoon lemon juice
- ½ cup almond flour
- 2 beets, peeled and grated
- 2 eggs, whisked
- ¼ cup tapioca flour
- 3 tablespoons olive oil

DIRECTIONS:

1. In a bowl, combine the garlic with the onions, scallions and the rest of the ingredients except the oil, stir well and shape medium fritters out of this mix.
2. Heat oil in a pan over medium-high heat, add the fritters, cook for 5 minutes on each side, arrange on a platter and serve.

NUTRITION: Calories 209 Fat 11.2 g Fiber 3 g Carbs 4.4 g Protein 4.8 g

181. White Bean Dip

Preparation Time: 10 minutes
Cooking Time: 0 minute
Servings: 4
INGREDIENTS:

- 15 ounces canned white beans, drained and rinsed
- 6 ounces canned artichoke hearts, drained and quartered
- 4 garlic cloves, minced
- 1 tablespoon basil, chopped
- 2 tablespoons olive oil
- Juice of ½ lemon
- Zest of ½ lemon, grated
- Salt and black pepper to the taste

DIRECTIONS:

1. In your food processor, combine the beans with the artichokes and the rest of the ingredients except the oil and pulse well.
2. Add the oil gradually, pulse the mix again, divide into cups and serve as a party dip.

NUTRITION: Calories 274 Fat 11.7 g Fiber 6.5 g Carbs 18.5 g Protein 16.5 g

182. Eggplant Dip

Preparation Time: 10 minutes
Cooking Time: 40 minutes
Servings: 4
INGREDIENTS:

- 1 eggplant, poked with a fork
- 2 tablespoons tahini paste
- 2 tablespoons lemon juice
- 2 garlic cloves, minced
- 1 tablespoon olive oil
- Salt and black pepper to the taste
- 1 tablespoon parsley, chopped

DIRECTIONS:

1. Put the eggplant in a roasting pan, bake at 400° F for 40 minutes, cool down, peel and transfer to your food processor.
2. Add the rest of the remaining ingredients except the parsley, pulse well, divide into small bowls and serve as an appetizer with the parsley sprinkled on top.

NUTRITION: Calories 121 Fat 4.3 g Fiber 1 g Carbs 1.4 g Protein 4.3 g

183. Bulgur Lamb Meatballs

Preparation Time: 10 minutes
Cooking Time: 15 minute
Servings: 6
INGREDIENTS:

- 1 and ½ cups Greek yogurt
- ½ teaspoon cumin, ground
- 1 cup cucumber, shredded
- ½ teaspoon garlic, minced
- A pinch of salt and black pepper
- 1 cup bulgur
- 2 cups water
- 1 pound lamb, ground
- ¼ cup parsley, chopped
- ¼ cup shallots, chopped
- ½ teaspoon allspice, ground
- ½ teaspoon cinnamon powder
- 1 tablespoon olive oil

DIRECTIONS:

1. Combine the bulgur with the water in a bowl, cover the bowl, leave aside for 10 minutes, drain and transfer to a bowl.
2. Add the meat, the yogurt and the rest of the ingredients except the oil, stir well and shape medium meatballs out of this mix.
3. Heat oil in a pan over medium-high heat, add the meatballs, cook them for 7 minutes on each side, arrange them all on a platter and serve as an appetizer.

NUTRITION: Calories 300 Fat 9.6 g Fiber 4.6 g Carbs 22.6 g Protein 6.6 g

184. Cucumber Bites

Preparation Time: 10 minutes
Cooking Time: 0 minutes
Servings: 12
INGREDIENTS:

- 1 English cucumber, sliced into 32 rounds
- 10 ounces hummus
- 16 cherry tomatoes, halved
- 1 tablespoon parsley, chopped
- 1 ounce feta cheese, crumbled

DIRECTIONS:

1. Spread the hummus on each cucumber round, divide the tomato halves on each, sprinkle the cheese and parsley on to and serve as an appetizer.

NUTRITION: Calories 162 Fat 3.4 g Fiber 2 g Carbs 6.4 g Protein 2.4 g

185. Stuffed Avocado

Preparation Time: 10 minutes
Cooking Time: 0 minute
Servings: 2
INGREDIENTS:

- 1 avocado, halved and pitted
- 10 ounces canned tuna, drained
- 2 tablespoons sun-dried tomatoes, chopped
- 1 and ½ tablespoon basil pesto
- 2 tablespoons black olives, pitted and chopped
- Salt and black pepper to the taste
- 2 teaspoons pine nuts, toasted and chopped
- 1 tablespoon basil, chopped

DIRECTIONS:

1. Combine the tuna with the sun-dried tomatoes in a bowl, and the rest of the ingredients except the avocado and stir.
2. Stuff the avocado halves with the tuna mix and serve as an appetizer.

NUTRITION: Calories 233 Fat 9 g Fiber 3.5 g Carbs 11.4 g Protein 5.6 g

186. Hummus with Ground Lamb

Preparation Time: 10 minutes
Cooking Time: 15 minute
Servings: 8
INGREDIENTS:

- 10 ounces hummus
- 12 ounces lamb meat, ground
- ½ cup pomegranate seeds
- ¼ cup parsley, chopped
- 1 tablespoon olive oil
- Pita chips for serving

DIRECTIONS:

1. Heat oil in a pan over medium-high heat, add the meat, and brown for 15 minutes stirring often.
2. Spread the hummus on a platter, spread the ground lamb all over, also spread the pomegranate seeds and the parsley and serve with pita chips as a snack.

NUTRITION: Calories 133 Fat 9.7 g Fiber 1.7 g Carbs 6.4 g Protein 5 g

187. Wrapped Plums

Preparation Time: 5 minutes
Cooking Time: 0 minutes
Servings: 8
INGREDIENTS:

- 2 ounces prosciutto, cut into 16 pieces
- 4 plums, quartered
- 1 tablespoon chives, chopped
- A pinch of red pepper flakes, crushed

DIRECTIONS:

1. Wrap each plum quarter in a prosciutto slice, arrange them all on a platter, sprinkle the chives and pepper flakes all over and serve.

NUTRITION: Calories 30 Fat 1 g Fiber 0 g Carbs 4 g Protein 2 g

188. Cucumber Sandwich Bites

Preparation Time: 5 minutes
Cooking Time: 0 minutes
Servings: 12
Ingredients:

- 1 cucumber, sliced
- 8 slices whole wheat bread
- 2 tablespoons cream cheese, soft
- 1 tablespoon chives, chopped
- ¼ cup avocado, peeled, pitted and mashed
- 1 teaspoon mustard
- Salt and black pepper to the taste

DIRECTIONS:

1. Spread the mashed avocado on each bread slice, also spread the rest of the ingredients except the cucumber slices. Divide the cucumber slices on the bread slices, cut each slice in thirds, arrange on a platter and serve as an appetizer.

NUTRITION: Calories 187 Fat 12.4 g Fiber 2.1 g Carbs 4.5 g Protein 8.2 g

189. Cucumber Rolls

Preparation Time: 5 minutes
Cooking Time: 0 minutes
Servings: 6
INGREDIENTS:

- 1 big cucumber, sliced lengthwise
- 1 tablespoon parsley, chopped
- 8 ounces canned tuna, drained and mashed
- Salt and black pepper to the taste
- 1 teaspoon lime juice

DIRECTIONS:

1. Arrange cucumber slices on a working surface, divide the rest of the ingredients, and roll.
2. Arrange all the rolls on a surface and serve as an appetizer.

NUTRITION: Calories 200 Fat 6 g Fiber 3.4 g Carbs 7.6 g Protein 3.5 g

190. Olives and Cheese Stuffed Tomatoes

Preparation Time: 10 minutes
Cooking Time: 0 minutes
Servings: 24
INGREDIENTS:

- 24 cherry tomatoes, top cut off and insides scooped out
- 2 tablespoons olive oil
- ¼ teaspoon red pepper flakes
- ½ cup feta cheese, crumbled
- 2 tablespoons black olive paste
- ¼ cup mint, torn

DIRECTIONS:

1. In a bowl, mix the olives paste with the rest of the ingredients except the cherry tomatoes and whisk well. Stuff the cherry tomatoes with this mix, arrange them all on a platter and serve as an appetizer.

NUTRITION: Calories 136 Fat 8.6 g Fiber 4.8 g Carbs 5.6 g Protein 5.1 g

191. Tomato Salsa

Preparation Time: 5 minutes
Cooking Time: 0 minutes
Servings: 6
INGREDIENTS:

- 1 garlic clove, minced
- 4 tablespoons olive oil
- 5 tomatoes, cubed
- 1 tablespoon balsamic vinegar
- ¼ cup basil, chopped
- 1 tablespoon parsley, chopped
- 1 tablespoon chives, chopped
- Salt and black pepper to the taste
- Pita chips for serving

DIRECTIONS:

1. Mix the tomatoes with the garlic in a bowl, and the rest of the ingredients except the pita chips, stir, divide into small cups and serve with the pita chips on the side.

NUTRITION: Calories 160 Fat 13.7 g Fiber 5.5 g Carbs 10.1 g Protein 2.2

192. Chili Mango and Watermelon Salsa

Preparation Time: 5 minutes
Cooking Time: 0 minutes
Servings: 12
INGREDIENTS:

- 1 red tomato, chopped
- Salt and black pepper to the taste
- 1 cup watermelon, seedless, peeled and cubed
- 1 red onion, chopped
- 2 mangos, peeled and chopped
- 2 chili peppers, chopped
- ¼ cup cilantro, chopped
- 3 tablespoons lime juice
- Pita chips for serving

DIRECTIONS:

1. In a bowl, mix the tomato with the watermelon, the onion and the rest of the ingredients except the pita chips and toss well. Divide the mix into small cups and serve with pita chips on the side.

NUTRITION: Calories 62 Fatg Fiber 1.3 g Carbs 3.9 g Protein 2.3 g

193. Creamy Spinach and Shallots Dip

Preparation Time: 10 minutes
Cooking Time: 0 minutes
Servings: 4
INGREDIENTS:

- 1 pound spinach, roughly chopped
- 2 shallots, chopped
- 2 tablespoons mint, chopped
- ¾ cup cream cheese, soft
- Salt and black pepper to the taste

DIRECTIONS:

1. Combine the spinach with the shallots and the rest of the ingredients in a blender,, and pulse well. Divide into small bowls and serve as a party dip.

NUTRITION: Calories 204 Fat 11.5 g Fiber 3.1 g Carbs 4.2 g Protein 5.9 g

194. Feta Artichoke Dip

Preparation Time: 10 minutes
Cooking Time: 30 minutes
Servings: 8
INGREDIENTS:

- 8 ounces artichoke hearts, drained and quartered
- ¾ cup basil, chopped
- ¾ cup green olives, pitted and chopped
- 1 cup parmesan cheese, grated
- 5 ounces feta cheese, crumbled

DIRECTIONS:

1. In your food processor, mix the artichokes with the basil and the rest of the ingredients, pulse well, and transfer to a baking dish.
2. Introduce in the oven, bake at 375° F for 30 minutes and serve as a party dip.

NUTRITION: Calories 186 Fat 12.4 g Fiber 0.9 g Carbs 2.6 g Protein 1.5 g

195. Avocado Dip

Preparation Time: 5 minutes
Cooking Time: 0 minutes
Servings: 8
INGREDIENTS:

- ½ cup heavy cream
- 1 green chili pepper, chopped
- Salt and pepper to the taste
- 4 avocados, pitted, peeled and chopped
- 1 cup cilantro, chopped
- ¼ cup lime juice

DIRECTIONS:

1. Pour the cream with the avocados and the rest of the ingredients in a blender, and pulse well. Divide the mix into bowls and serve cold as a party dip.

NUTRITION: Calories 200 Fat 14.5 g Fiber 3.8 g Carbs 8.1 g Protein 7.6 g

196. Goat Cheese and Chives Spread

Preparation Time: 10 minutes
Cooking Time: 0 minute
Servings: 4
INGREDIENTS:

- 2 ounces goat cheese, crumbled
- ¾ cup sour cream
- 2 tablespoons chives, chopped
- 1 tablespoon lemon juice
- Salt and black pepper to the taste
- 2 tablespoons extra virgin olive oil

DIRECTIONS:

1. Mix the goat cheese with the cream and the rest of the ingredients in a bowl, and whisk really well. Keep in the fridge for 10 minutes and serve as a party spread.

NUTRITION: Calories 220 Fat 11.5 g Fiber 4.8 g Carbs 8.9 g Protein 5.6 g

DESSERTS

197. Chocolate Bars

Preparation Time: 10 minutes
Cooking Time: 20 minutes
Servings: 16
INGREDIENTS:

- 15 oz cream cheese, softened
- 15 oz unsweetened dark chocolate
- 1 tsp vanilla
- 10 drops liquid stevia

DIRECTIONS:

1. Grease 8-inch square dish and set aside.
2. In a saucepan dissolve chocolate over low heat.
3. Add stevia and vanilla and stir well.
4. Remove pan from heat and set aside.
5. Add cream cheese into the blender and blend until smooth.
6. Add melted chocolate mixture into the cream cheese and blend until just combined.
7. Transfer mixture into the prepared dish and spread evenly and place in the refrigerator until firm.
8. Slice and serve.

NUTRITION: Calories: 230 Fat: 24 g Carbs: 7.5 g Sugar: 0.1 g Protein: 6 g Cholesterol: 29 mg

198. Blueberry Muffins

Preparation Time: 15 minutes
Cooking Time: 35 minutes
Servings: 12
INGREDIENTS:

- 2 eggs
- 1/2 cup fresh blueberries
- 1 cup heavy cream
- 2 cups almond flour
- 1/4 tsp lemon zest
- 1/2 tsp lemon extract
- 1 tsp baking powder
- 5 drops stevia
- 1/4 cup butter, melted

DIRECTIONS:

1. heat the cooker to 350 F. Line muffin tin with cupcake liners and set aside.
2. Add eggs into the bowl and whisk until mix.
3. Add remaining ingredients and mix to combine.
4. Pour mixture into the prepared muffin tin and bake for 25 minutes.
5. Serve and enjoy.

NUTRITION: Calories: 190 Fat: 17 g Carbs: 5 g Sugar: 1 g Protein: 5 g Cholesterol: 55 mg

199. Chia Pudding

Preparation Time: 20 minutes
Cooking Time: 0 minutes
Servings: 2
INGREDIENTS:

- 4 tbsp chia seeds
- 1 cup unsweetened coconut milk
- 1/2 cup raspberries

DIRECTIONS:

1. Add raspberry and coconut milk into a blender and blend until smooth.
2. Pour mixture into the glass jar.
3. Add chia seeds in a jar and stir well.
4. Seal the jar with a lid and shake well and place in the refrigerator for 3 hours.
5. Serve chilled and enjoy.

NUTRITION: Calories: 360 Fat: 33 g Carbs: 13 g Sugar: 5 g Protein: 6 g Cholesterol: 0 mg

200. Avocado Pudding

Preparation Time: 20 minutes
Cooking Time: 0 minutes
Servings: 8
INGREDIENTS:

- 2 ripe avocados, pitted and cut into pieces
- 1 tbsp fresh lime juice
- 14 oz can coconut milk
- 2 tsp liquid stevia
- 2 tsp vanilla

DIRECTIONS:

1. Inside the blender Add all ingredients and blend until smooth.
2. Serve immediately and enjoy.

NUTRITION: Calories: 317 Fat: 30 g Carbs: 9 g Sugar: 0.5 g Protein: 3 g Cholesterol: 0 mg

201. Delicious Brownie Bites

Preparation Time: 20 minutes
Cooking Time: 0 minutes
Servings: 13
INGREDIENTS:

- 1/4 cup unsweetened chocolate chips
- 1/4 cup unsweetened cocoa powder
- 1 cup pecans, chopped
- 1/2 cup almond butter
- 1/2 tsp vanilla
- 1/4 cup monk fruit sweetener
- 1/8 tsp pink salt

DIRECTIONS:

1. Add pecans, sweetener, vanilla, almond butter, cocoa powder, and salt into the food processor and process until well combined.
2. Transfer brownie mixture into the large bowl. Add chocolate chips and fold well.
3. Make small round shape balls from brownie mixture and place onto a baking tray.
4. Place in the freezer for 20 minutes.
5. Serve and enjoy.

NUTRITION: Calories: 108 Fat: 9 g Carbs: 4 g Sugar: 1 g Protein: 2 g Cholesterol: 0 mg

202. Pumpkin Balls

Preparation Time: 15 minutes
Cooking Time: 0 minutes
Servings: 18
INGREDIENTS:

- 1 cup almond butter
- 5 drops liquid stevia
- 2 tbsp coconut flour
- 2 tbsp pumpkin puree
- 1 tsp pumpkin pie spice

DIRECTIONS:

1. Mix together pumpkin puree in a large bowl, and almond butter until well combined.
2. Add liquid stevia, pumpkin pie spice, and coconut flour and mix well.
3. Make small balls from mixture and place onto a baking tray.
4. Place in the freezer for 1 hour.
5. Serve and enjoy.

NUTRITION: Calories: 96 Fat: 8 g Carbs: 4 g Sugar: 1 g Protein: 2 g Cholesterol: 0 mg

203. Smooth Peanut Butter Cream

Preparation Time: 10 minutes
Cooking Time: 0 minutes
Servings: 8
INGREDIENTS:

- 1/4 cup peanut butter
- 4 overripe bananas, chopped
- 1/3 cup cocoa powder
- 1/4 tsp vanilla extract
- 1/8 tsp salt

DIRECTIONS:

1. In the blender add all the listed ingredients and blend until smooth.
2. Serve immediately and enjoy.

NUTRITION: Calories: 101 Fat: 5 g Carbs: 14 g Sugar: 7 g Protein: 3 g Cholesterol: 0 mg

204. Vanilla Avocado Popsicles

Preparation Time: 20 minutes
Cooking Time: 0 minutes
Servings: 6
INGREDIENTS:

- 2 avocadoes
- 1 tsp vanilla
- 1 cup almond milk
- 1 tsp liquid stevia
- 1/2 cup unsweetened cocoa powder

DIRECTIONS:

1. In the blender add all the listed ingredients and blend smoothly.
2. Pour blended mixture into the Popsicle molds and place in the freezer until set.
3. Serve and enjoy.

NUTRITION: Calories: 130 Fat: 12 g Carbs: 7 g Sugar: 1 g Protein: 3 g Cholesterol: 0 mg

205. Chocolate Popsicle

Preparation Time: 20 minutes
Cooking Time: 10 minutes
Servings: 6
INGREDIENTS:

- 4 oz unsweetened chocolate, chopped
- 6 drops liquid stevia
- 1 1/2 cups heavy cream

DIRECTIONS:

1. Add heavy cream into the microwave-safe bowl and microwave until just begins the boiling.
2. Add chocolate into the heavy cream and set aside for 5 minutes.
3. Add liquid stevia into the heavy cream mixture and stir until chocolate is melted.
4. Pour mixture into the Popsicle molds and place in freezer for 4 hours or until set.
5. Serve and enjoy.

NUTRITION: Calories: 198 Fat: 21 g Carbs: 6 g Sugar: 0.2 g Protein: 3 g Cholesterol: 41 mg

206. Raspberry Ice Cream

Preparation Time: 10 minutes
Cooking Time: 0 minutes
Servings: 2
INGREDIENTS:

- 1 cup frozen raspberries
- 1/2 cup heavy cream
- 1/8 tsp stevia powder

DIRECTIONS:

1. Blend all the listed ingredients in a blender until smooth.
2. Serve immediately and enjoy.

NUTRITION: Calories: 144 Fat: 11 g Carbs: 10 g Sugar: 4 g Protein: 2 g Cholesterol: 41 mg

207. Chocolate Frosty

Preparation Time: 20 minutes
Cooking Time: 0 minutes
Servings: 4
INGREDIENTS:

- 2 tbsp unsweetened cocoa powder
- 1 cup heavy whipping cream
- 1 tbsp almond butter
- 5 drops liquid stevia
- 1 tsp vanilla

DIRECTIONS:

1. Add cream into the medium bowl and beat using the hand mixer for 5 minutes.
2. Add remaining ingredients and blend until thick cream form.
3. Pour in serving bowls and place them in the freezer for 30 minutes.
4. Serve and enjoy.

NUTRITION: Calories: 137 Fat: 13 g Carbs: 3 g Sugar: 0.5 g Protein: 2 g Cholesterol: 41 mg

208. Chocolate Almond Butter Brownie

Preparation Time: 10 minutes
Cooking Time: 16 minutes
Servings: 4
INGREDIENTS:

- 1 cup bananas, overripe
- 1/2 cup almond butter, melted
- 1 scoop protein powder
- 2 tbsp unsweetened cocoa powder

DIRECTIONS:

1. Preheat the air fryer to 325 F. Grease air fryer baking pan and set aside.
2. Blend all ingredients in a blender until smooth.
3. Pour batter into the prepared pan and place in the air fryer basket and cook for 16 minutes.
4. Serve and enjoy.

NUTRITION: Calories: 82 Fat: 2 g Carbs: 11 g Sugar: 5 g Protein: 7 g Cholesterol: 16 mg

209. Peanut Butter Fudge

Preparation Time: 10 minutes
Cooking Time: 10 minutes
Servings: 20
INGREDIENTS:

- 1/4 cup almonds, toasted and chopped
- 12 oz smooth peanut butter
- 15 drops liquid stevia
- 3 tbsp coconut oil
- 4 tbsp coconut cream
- Pinch of salt

DIRECTIONS:

1. Line baking tray with parchment paper.
2. Melt coconut oil in a pan over low heat. Add peanut butter, coconut cream, stevia, and salt in a saucepan. Stir well.
3. Pour fudge mixture into the prepared baking tray and sprinkle chopped almonds on top.
4. Place the tray in the refrigerator for 1 hour or until set.
5. Slice and serve.

NUTRITION: Calories: 131 Fat: 12 g Carbs: 4 g Sugar: 2 g Protein: 5 g Cholesterol: 0 mg

210. Almond Butter Fudge

Preparation Time: 10 minutes
Cooking Time: 10 minutes
Servings: 18
INGREDIENTS:

- 3/4 cup creamy almond butter
- 1 1/2 cups unsweetened chocolate chips

DIRECTIONS:

1. Line 8*4-inch pan with parchment paper and set aside.
2. Add chocolate chips and almond butter into the double boiler and cook over medium heat until the chocolate-butter mixture is melted. Stir well.
3. place mixture into the prepared pan and place in the freezer until set.
4. Slice and serve.

NUTRITION: Calories: 197 Fat: 16 g Carbs: 7 g Sugar: 1 g Protein: 4 g Cholesterol: 0 mg

CPSIA information can be obtained
at www.ICGtesting.com
Printed in the USA
BVHW050621080221
599618BV00011B/458

9 781649 847423